MAKE IT SAFE!

A Family Caregiver's Home Safety Assessment Guide for Supporting Elders@Home

RAE A. STONEHOUSE

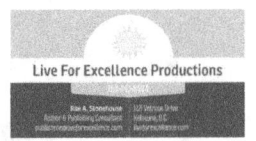

Copyright © 2020 by Rae A. Stonehouse

All rights reserved.

No part of this book may be reproduced in any form or by any electronic or mechanical means, including information storage and retrieval systems, without written permission from the author, except for the use of brief quotations in a book review.

Fair Use Notice: This publication contains copyrighted material the use of which has not been specifically authorized by the copyright owner and is readily found on the Internet. In each case the content's source has been identified. The copyright to the content remains with the original author and source of the content and is not included in the copyright ascertained by the Author, Rae A. Stonehouse.

Disclaimer: The publisher and the author are providing this book and its contents on "as is" basis and make no representations or warranties of any kind with respect to this book or its contents. The publisher and the author disclaim all such representations and warranties, including but not limited to warranties of healthcare for a particular purpose. In addition, the publisher and author assume no responsibility for errors, inaccuracies, omissions, or any other inconsistencies herein

Do your own research: The content of this book is intended to be used and must be used for informational purposes only. It is very important to do your own assessments before investing in renovations or purchasing safety equipment based on your own personal circumstances. You should independently research and verify any information provided in this book and wish to act upon.

This publication is meant as a source of valuable information for the reader, however it is not meant as a substitute for direct expert assistance. If such level of assistance is required, the services of a competent professional should be sought.

The publisher and the author make no guarantees concerning the level of success you may experience by following the advice and strategies contained in this book and you accept the results will differ with each individual.

E-book - ISBN: 978-1-7771565-2-7
Print - ISBN: 978-1-7771565-3-4
Large Print - ISBN - 978-1-7771565-4-1
Companion Workbook - ISBN 978-1-7771565-5-8

Live For Excellence Productions
1221 Velrose Drive
Kelowna, B.C., Canada
V1X6R7
https://liveforexcellence.com

Created with Vellum

SECTION ONE: ELDERCARE@HOME OVERVIEW

INTRODUCTION

It is often said "it takes a village to raise a child." The same can be said about helping an elder age at home. Perhaps not a village, but certainly a family.

With advancements in modern medicine, our aging population, on the whole, is living longer.

While many elders are living longer, they are not necessarily living better. Many are living with complex chronic medical conditions, requiring ongoing monitoring and support.

Those who would've succumbed to acute or chronic diseases and ailments in the past are continuing to live longer lives due to the benefits of ongoing medication.

We can't generalize or lump all seniors or elderly people into a one-size-fits-all category. Many seniors remain active, vibrant and mentally alert into their 90s. Yet, others seem old in their early 60s.

Caregiving at home has proven its value in offsetting the high costs of in-facility healthcare, and at the same time, improving the quality of life for many elders. However, educational training and support for caregivers has been in short supply.

Traditionally, in many cultures, the role of caring for and supporting aging parents has fallen to an unmarried daughter.

The caregiving role has changed over the years with many men stepping into the role. There is a current trend of younger people in their late teens and early 20s taking on the caretaking role for their parents who may be aging or suffering from chronic illnesses.

Taking on the role of supporting an elder living independently in the community or living with your family in your home can be an immense and daunting responsibility.

Our formal education and training haven't prepared us to take on the role of caregiver. So how do we do it?

The focus of this book is to help you as a family caregiver create a safe living space and conditions to support an elder living semi-independently in the community or adapting your family household to support an elder as a member of your family.

Make it Safe! A Family Caregivers Home Safety Assessment Guide for Supporting Elders@Home started as a module focusing on elderly safety in the **Elder@Home Awareness Program** which I had been contracted as a consultant to create for a local non-profit organization.

As a recently retired Registered Nurse of over 40 years, I have worked predominantly in the field of mental health/psychiatry. I have experience working with the elderly in senior's facilities, psychogeriatric units, mental health facilities and in the community.

Over the years I've taught various healthcare programs to adults in post-secondary school settings.

While working as a Registered Nurse I have been actively involved with Occupational Health & Safety in my workplaces. That experience has been beneficial in developing my skills to take an analytical look at a home's potential safety hazards and to provide strategies to rectify those hazards to make it safe for an elder to live there.

As an aside, in developing this safety program, it has created a massive To Do list of items I need to complete in my own home as my wife and I hope to age in place.

As an author and creator of several self-help books and on-line courses, I take a systematic approach to exploring a specific subject.

We begin with an overview of home safety. We look at a method of completing an assessment of the home's safety status and develop strategies to rectify the problems or hazards to make the home safe.

There is a lot of information on the Internet right now about how to make the home safe for an elder. The information provided can be well meaning, yet falls short of providing the rationale behind their safety tip or considerations you might need to make before deciding on your course of action.

Make it Safe! A Family Caregivers Home Safety Assessment Guide for Supporting Elders@Home is a compilation of readily available safety tips, adds to them and takes them to the next level. This is a book meant to be read, and then put into action. A downloadable home safety inspection sheet is provided so you can complete an elder's home inspection, or yours for that matter.

There is also a companion workbook to this book entitled **Make it Safe! A Family Caregivers Home Safety Assessment Guide for Supporting Elders@Home - Companion Workbook** available that may make your task a little easier.

Note: Links to additional resources and sources of the content have been included throughout the book. Websites tend to change frequently and the link that worked when the book was published, may no longer work. If you find a link that doesn't work, I would suggest copying the url link and pasting it into a Google search bar. In most cases it should provide you access to the resource. Sorry for the inconvenience.

After our introduction of home safety concerns, we move on to an overview of general home safety matters. We systematically work our way through the home, focusing on specific rooms or areas where we are provided with **Safety Assessment Questions** to answer.

Many of the safety assessment questions are accompanied by **Considerations** to help you decide your course of action as well as the **Rationale** behind the question. That is, why is it important and why do you need to care about this potential problem. Each question is backed up with **Action Items** to suggest what you can or need to do to solve the problem and make it safe for you, your family and the elder.

Throughout the book I have provided **[Author's Comments]** sharing anecdotes from my personal experience to illustrate various points. In addition, I've included **Make it Safe TIPs** to draw attention to important suggestions.

After we work our way through the home, we look at three chapters focusing on electrical safety, fire safety and home use of medical devices. We complete this section on home safety by looking at elderly driving concerns and providing guidance for ongoing support and follow-up for your aging at home elder.

In our final section, Section Three, we look at maintaining your elder's health and wellbeing as they successfully age at home. This is your ongoing follow-up stage.

We also look at day-to-day healthcare supervision, medication management safety, emergency preparedness and finish with an exploration of scams targeting the elderly.

We start our eldercare safety journey in the next chapter looking at an overview of the Caregiver role.

Rae A. Stonehouse, Author

June 2020

OVERVIEW OF THE FAMILY CAREGIVER ROLE

The Caregiving Journey

In Canada alone, more than eight million people—or 28% of the population aged 15 and over—provide care to older adult family members or friends, and the numbers will continue to climb as the proportion of older adults continues to rise. Eighty percent of older adults and people with long-term health issues are cared for at home by family and friends.

CAREGIVING IS ONE OF THE GREATEST GIFTS WE CAN PROVIDE A loved one and can also be a very rewarding experience. But it can also involve many challenges to the health, well-being and financial security of caregivers.

As a caregiver, it is important to talk to family, friends, other caregivers and professionals to share information and find out about local supports and services. Accept offers of help and arrange for respite whenever and however you can. While caring for a loved one may be a top priority for you, it is also important to take care of your own health and well-being.

Source: McMaster Optimal Aging Portal https://www.mcmasteroptimalaging.org/hitting-the-headlines/detail/hitting-the-headlines/2019/04/02/the-rewards-and-challenges-that-come-with-caregiving

The caregiving journey can look different for everyone. Perhaps a few months after a loved one has had surgical procedure, or caregiving can be a role somebody takes on for several years supporting their loved one who has chronic conditions. It can even last decades for someone who cares for a loved one with Parkinson's or some type of dementia, such as Alzheimer's disease.

DETERMINING WHEN A CARE CHANGE IS NEEDED

A challenge many families experience is deciding when an elderly family member or loved one requires a change in their living accommodations.

There are two general categories: How to know when it is time to transition from independence in the home and when it is time to move from home to a care facility.

Independence to Support in the Home:

Mental:

• Forgetfulness that impacts daily life

• Accidents in the kitchen such as the stove being left on e.g. scorched pots and pans

• Losing track of medications

• Missing doctor's appointments and social engagements

• Mail and bills are piling up

Emotional and Social:

- Reluctance to leave the house (might be due to cognitive impairment, mobility limitations or transportation issues.)

- Withdrawing from social interactions (might be a sign of depression)

Physical and Medical:

- Losing interest in meals or cooking. Could be medical issues like arthritis that are preventing them from cooking.

- Declining driving skills

- Declining personal hygiene. Perhaps they are afraid of using the bathtub or showering due to a fear of falling.

- If they always had a clean and tidy home and now it is unkempt, it may be a sign something else is going on.

Home to Facility:

It can be a difficult decision to make. Some adult children have promised their parent they will never move them to a facility, then they are challenged to follow through on that promise.

Here are some general indicators to determine when it is time to move from a home to a facility setting or a community setting:

- Refusal to accept professional help at home

- Care needs are beyond level of care available in the home. Maybe they have a medical condition, or the layout of the home is not conducive to their safety or the home environment can't be modified to meet their needs.

- For those with dementia or Alzheimer's, if behavioral symptoms are too much to manage at home. The disease symptoms could put the caregiver or the care recipient in danger.

- Cost for 24-hour care in the home is outside of financial ability to pay for services. Even if a family creates a schedule and supplements with outside help, it may be more financially feasible to consider moving them into a care facility.

Every situation is different, and this list doesn't cover all situations. The decision should involve the elder and any family member who wants to be part of the decision-making process.

IN OUR NEXT SECTION, SECTION TWO, WE LOOK AT ASSESSING safety hazards in different areas of the elder's home or living accommodations.

SECTION TWO: HOME SAFETY

HOME SAFETY OVERVIEW

I f you are a parent, you will probably remember what it was like to make your home safe for your children.

MANY OF THE SAME PRINCIPLES APPLY WHEN MAKING YOUR HOME safe for elders. Whereas, with children you are usually protecting them from accessing something that could be hazardous and could cause them harm, when making the home safe for elders, you will also be thinking about <u>accessibility</u>, <u>accommodating decreased mobility</u> and <u>memory deficits</u>.

At the same time, you need to be able to support the elder in maintaining their independence as long as you can and as long as they are able.

IN THIS SECTION WE LOOK AT MAKING YOUR HOME SAFER FOR AN elder to reside with you or making adaptations to the elder's current home, allowing them to live independently, with your support.

Throughout the book I use the terms 'elder', 'senior' and 'loved one' interchangeably. While this book is written from the perspective of helping an older person to live safely either independently or semi-independently in their own home, or yours, the same safety principles apply to caring for someone who is not elderly.

To do so, we will be drawing from the field of <u>personal safety</u> as a way to organize ourselves.

Introducing the **3 As of Personal safety**... <u>Awareness, Assessment and Action.</u>

Awareness: As we go about the activities of our daily life, we likely encounter many situations or conditions that are hazardous. Hopefully, we have learned how to avoid or prevent negative results from these hazards.

This is <u>your</u> awareness. You realize a particular situation could be hazardous to you so you take avoidant or corrective actions to prevent harm or injury.

This section on home safety will serve to raise your awareness on how the safety needs of an elder can be greater than what we may be used to.

I would suspect upon completion of this book you will identify hazards in your home needing rectifying for the benefit of your entire family, not just an elderly person as I did when developing this program.

Assessment: At a basic level, assessment is where you will be doing a walk-about inspection of the elder's living environment.

Much the same as a home inspector would do an investigation of a home you were considering purchasing... letting you know what is right or wrong with the house, you will be conducting a safety inspection of the elder's home.

As we work our way through the book, we will be exploring a collection of safety-related questions, focusing on different areas of the home.

The chapters are organized in main areas common to most homes and suggestions are provided to the questions posed.

As you work your way through the content, you will notice there are specific hazards common to many areas of the home. They will be identified in the chapter you are reading. To draw attention to their importance, some will have their own specific chapter examples: Fire Safety and Electrical Safety.

If you can think of a safety concern we missed, please let us know so we can share with others.

Home Safety Assessment Form: I have created a set of question sheets you can print and carry with you to complete your inspection. You can access them and download them at https//BookHip.com/SXGMBT.

It can be helpful to use a clipboard when you are performing your safety inspection.

Action: It doesn't help anybody if you identify a hazard and don't do anything to resolve it.

Resolving a problem may mean taking a piece of equipment such as a toaster with a faulty cord out of service, repairing a hazard or perhaps undergoing a major renovation to accommodate the elder's needs.

Create a Safety Upgrade Budget.

There are several steps to creating a budget for safety upgrades.

Some fixes you may be able to do fairly quickly. Others may take time to organize and to raise the funds to pay for the upgrades.

Once you identify a safety hazard needing improving, you need to research the options available and determine a cost.

As well, are you able to make the improvements yourself, or will you require a professional tradesperson to make the improvements? This will affect the costs involved in the home improvement.

While we complete our safety inspection, we will keep track of items that may require a budget to rectify.

Depending on where you live, there may be government or NGO (non-government organizations) funds you could access to offset the costs of home safety improvements.

In the next chapter we start our home inspection inside the home. We look in detail at specific hazards and provide commentary on further considerations.

As we work our way through our home inspection we also look at safety devices that can be purchased to solve safety problems or to facilitate the elder's continued level of functioning.

Please note we are not recommending specific products and you should undertake your due dilligence before purchasing any product and putting it into service.

HOME SAFETY - INDOORS
GENERAL

In this chapter we look at general areas of safety concern within the home. We expand upon many of them in upcoming chapters.

Action: Do a walk about assessment

Take the **Home Safety Assessment Form** with you and do a walk about inspection of the inside of the elder's home.

If the elder lives with you, you could very well be conducting an assessment of your own home, however with a different set of eyes i.e. with the safety of an elder in mind.

This section of the book is organized by offering you a series of **Safety Assessment Questions.**

We follow along with the <u>**3 A's of Personal Safety**</u> formula discussed in the previous chapter.

Many of the questions present you with the **Rationale** behind the question i.e. the logic or reason behind the assessment question.

Some questions will also offer you **Considerations** to help you make your decision as to determining your next step.

Finally, **Action Items** will be provided to guide you to possible solutions for the hazards you have identified.

If you see a safety hazard, make it safe as soon as possible.

If you see a safety hazard, fix it as soon as possible. It may be a simple fix of taking a defective appliance out of service. Other fixes may take time and/or need to be budgeted for.

As you work your way through the home inspection, make note of items you will need to follow-up on resolving or investigating further.

There are a lot of items in this inspection and it can be easy to want to start solving problems before you complete your assessment.

Stay the course. Complete your home assessment, then create your action plan to resolve items identified. Perhaps solving the easy ones first might be a good start.

Safety Assessment Question: Is house clean & tidy?

Considerations: Is the home reasonably clean and tidy? Is the house stocked with dish soap, laundry soap and other cleaning supplies?

Action Item: if the home isn't tidy, make note of the fact and return to this item upon completion of your assessment. At that time make a list of areas needing tidying and create a list of cleaning supplies you may need to purchase.

Safety Assessment Question: Is the home safe for a professional caregiver to visit the home?

Rationale: Professional caregivers are trained to consider their own health and safety first. If the home presents a potential hazard to their personal safety, they may deny service until the hazard has been rectified.

If the elder is a smoker, they may be required to refrain from smoking for a specific amount of time to reduce the hazards of second-hand smoke to the caregiver.

Action Item: If the elder requires the services of a professional caregiver who provides services within the elder's home, speak to the caregiver about their requirements and/or health & safety needs.

Safety Assessment Question: Are emergency numbers posted?

Considerations: Emergency numbers include: poison control, physicians, most responsible family member, 911 for police, fire or ambulance, an involved neighbor, etc.

Action Items:

- If an Emergency Number List hasn't been created, make one.
- Post the list in an easily accessible location such as on the refrigerator.

Safety Assessment Question: Is there a designated danger zone in the home to store hazardous chemicals or products?

Rationale: People with dementia forget the purpose of things and how to use them. They may think wiper fluid is juice or be unaware that the grill is hot.

Action Items:

1. Designate a danger zone.
2. To make the home safer, turn the garage, workroom, closet, outdoor shed, recycled TV armoire or a large cabinet into a storage place for:

- cleaning products
- bleach
- mothballs
- insecticide
- paint, turpentine, stain
- sharp knives, scissors, box cutters, blades
- alcohol
- tobacco products, including chewing tobacco
- hand and power tools

1. Better still, remove these products completely from the home and find alternative storage. You could then bring them with you when you visited the home if you required them.
2. Install key or combination locks on rooms and other storage places containing potentially dangerous items. In addition, use childproof doorknob covers or cabinet locks.

~

Safety Assessment Question: Is there good lighting in stairways & hallways?

Considerations: Make home lighting brighter but prevent glare.

Action Item: Provide good lighting where required.

Safety Assessment Question: Does every room have proper lighting, including walk-in closets?

Action Items:

1. Ensure every room has proper lighting, including walk-in closets. Use a nightlight to make it easy to see at night. Battery operated nightlights are available for areas without electrical access.
2. Place a light (such as a lamp) close to the bed and make sure the elder can reach it easily.
3. Extra lamps: consider models that turn on and off with a touch.

Safety Assessment Question: Are light switches installed at the top and bottom of staircases?

Action Item: If not present, install light switches at the top and bottom of your staircases.

Safety Assessment Question: Are bookshelves anchored to walls to prevent toppling over?

Action Item: Ensure bookshelves are anchored to walls. Heavy duty anti-tip furniture straps are readily available for purchase at your local hardware store.

Safety Assessment Questions: Is a smoke and carbon monoxide detector present?

Do the detectors work?

When were the batteries last changed?

How often are the batteries changed and by whom?

Rationale: Carbon monoxide is a deadly, odorless, colorless gas—you cannot smell it or see it. Having a working carbon monoxide detector is crucial to elder safety! And to your own...

Action Item: If your smoke or carbon monoxide detectors are more than 10 years old, it's time to replace them!

Safety Assessment Question: Are there any wheeled swivel chairs in the home?

Rationale: Wheeled swivel chairs can be a danger to an elderly person. The chair can easily move out from under them when they attempt to sit or get up from.

Action Item: If practical, remove the wheels from the chair.

Or remove from the home or keep in a room the elder doesn't have access to.

Safety Assessment Question: Do bedrooms or bathrooms have locks that can be released should an elder lock themselves in?

Rationale: Cabinet locks, door guardians, and refrigerator locks can prevent access to storage areas or exits from the house to discourage wandering or exploring, which might end badly.

Action Items:

1. Remove locks from bedroom and bathroom doors so you can get in quickly, should the elder fall.
2. Switch out standard doorknobs for lever handles.

Safety Assessment Question: Are doorways and halls wide enough for an elder to navigate with a wheelchair or walker?

Action Item: If required: offset door hinges to make room for a wheelchair, walker or two people walking side by side.

Safety Assessment Question: Are cordless phones within easy reach of the elder?

Action Item: Have a cordless phone at the elder's home and keep it within easy reach, to prevent having to rush to answer when the phone rings.

Consideration: If you are purchasing new cordless phones, consider a multi-unit set. This will allow you to have one unit in the charger which you can easily swap out with one with a reduced power charge whenever you visit the elder's home.

Safety Assessment Questions: Is the furniture stable?

Do chairs wobble when sat in?

Are chair arms, seat cushions, chair backs, etc. all in good condition?

Action Items:

1. Ensure all furniture an elder might use in their daily activity is safe for use. If not, either repair the item or remove from service.
2. Discard or donate old furniture.

Safety Assessment Question: Are furniture cushion levels at the right level to allow the elder to easily sit down?

Action Item: Use firm foam cushions to raise the height of furniture.

Safety Assessment Question: Are electrical cords or cables exposed in a way that could be a trip hazard?

Action Item: Avoid stretching extension cords across the floor.

Safety Assessment Question: Are there any barriers to creating a safe home?

Safety Assessment Question: Are bed rails required for the elder sleeping safety?

Consideration: If already in place, are they being used safely & correctly?

Safety Assessment Question: Is the elder's bed at a level that allows them to place their feet on the floor when attempting to stand up from the bed?

Consideration: Pay attention to the height of the elder's bed: if their feet can't touch the floor while sitting on the bed, it means their bed is too high.

Action Items:

1. Try lowering the bed by removing the box spring.
2. Similarly, if their knees are higher than their hips while sitting, it means the bed is too low. In this case, try adding a box spring.

Safety Assessment Question: Is the elder's clothing safe?

Consideration: Does the elder wear clothing that may become a hazard?

Examples: loose sleeves can become entangled in appliances or a fire hazard when cooking on the stove, ties can become caught in household appliances.

Action Items:

1. Observe the clothing the elder wears when cooking.

2. If the sleeves or other aspect of the clothing appears to be hazardous, suggest to the elder to change their clothing to something safer.

Safety Assessment Question: Does the home have an adequate heating system or does the elder use the stove or oven to provide heat?

Consideration: Heat the home safely – do not use an oven as a heating source, under any circumstance.

Action Item: Encourage the elder to turn off all portable heaters if and when they leave the home.

Safety Assessment Question: Have you developed an escape route in case of fire and a fire safety plan?

Action Item: We discuss this in detail in an upcoming chapter on fire safety.

Safety Assessment Question: If the elder uses a space heater, is it placed well away from flammable substances and materials?

Action Item: We also discuss this in detail in an upcoming chapter on fire safety.

Safety Assessment Question: Is there any evidence of leaks in the home as evidenced by water stains on a ceiling or an interior wall?

Rationale: Water stains on a ceiling or actively dripping water can indicate a leaky roof or perhaps a problem with a leaky toilet, bathtub or shower.

Action Items:

1. Check for leaks in the roof around windows and doors.
2. Replace broken windows, which can allow for cold air to enter the room.

3. If water leakage and damage is due to a plumbing leak, have a qualified plumber solve the problem.

[Author's Comments] I've described my family's home elsewhere in this book as being a three-level, split level home.

On one occasion, my mother had been sitting in her favorite chair in the living room watching television. She felt a sudden urge to check on something in the kitchen.

Upon going down the short three-step staircase to the kitchen, she heard a loud, almost deafening sound [her words].

Looking back up into the living room, all she could see was a cloud of dust. A four by eight feet section of the ceiling had collapsed, landing directly on where she had been sitting in her chair only moments before.

Was it divine intervention? Clairvoyance, perhaps? Whatever it was saved her life.

Upon investigation she found the plaster ceiling had given way, bringing down the plaster, the wooden lath and the water sodden fiberglass insulation.

When my parents had a roof repairman, take a look at the mess, they were advised the cause of the problem had been a leak, high up on the roof, causing water to drip down and pool directly above where my mother sat. He estimated that with the water soaked insulation there was probably a couple thousand pounds of weight in what came tumbling down.

My mother told me there had been a small water stain on the ceiling above where she sat, however they didn't do anything about it as they also had one in the kitchen for years from a toilet directly above it.

It goes to show that complacence, or procrastination to repair a problem can have dire consequences.

Safety Assessment Question: Do you have a first aid kit and know where it is?

Action Item: Is the first aid kit checked regularly to ensure supplies are replenished?

Miscellaneous Safety Measures:

In the next part of this chapter we look at a collection of miscellaneous safety measures to help an elder live safely in our home or in their own home.

Cover furniture corners to prevent injuries if you accidentally bump into them.

Water Heater Temperature

Rationale: As we age, our skin and body fat can become thinner. This can cause an elder to bruise and burn easier than a younger person.

Action Item: If you have a water boiler/hot water heater, don't set the thermostat to "Hot". Instead, use the "Medium" setting to avoid burns or scalding.

[Author's Comments:] I would suggest caution even if you have set your water heater's thermostat to Medium.

When a large amount of hot water is used, such as when someone takes a bath, the water in the heater is replaced with cold water. This new, cold water is then heated.

It could mean the next person taking a bath could be exposed to very hot water.

I reduced our family hot water heater to the Medium setting so my grandchild wouldn't be scalded, only to find it was pumping out very hot water after the first bath.

I'm glad the water heater is efficient, but I remain cautious about the possibilities of scalds and have cautioned my family members.

Mixing cleaning products:

Do not mix cleaning products together–some substances may be extremely dangerous when combined.

Rationale: For example, one of the most common hazards occurs when chlorine bleach is mixed with ammonia or acids.

The combination of ammonia and bleach produces dangerous chlorine gas, which in small doses can cause irritation to the eyes, skin and respiratory tract.

In large doses, it can kill. Chlorine gas, also known as mustard gas, was actually used in WWI & WWII.

[Author's Comments] One of my coworkers shared a personal story with me. She was not aware of the dangers of mixing chlorine bleach and ammonia.

She related she had mixed up a batch of solution to do some extra-strength household cleaning. She told me it resulted in burning eyes, a burnt feeling in her nose and nasal passages as well as causing her eyebrows to fall off.

She was lucky she wasn't killed.

Controls & switches that are reachable from a wheelchair or bed:

Action Item: If possible, are you able to relocate controls and switches so they are reachable from a wheelchair or bed?

Laundry facilities on first floor:

Rationale: Many older homes have a laundry area set up in the basement. Having to go up and down the basement steps repeatedly can be troublesome for an elder with mobility problems.

There can also be other safety concerns inherent with a basement laundry room such as inadequate lighting, dampness/wetness, flooring surface hazards.

[Author's Comments] My aging mother suffered from emphysema and other unspecified breathing problems. Her basement housed an oil-burning furnace and an oil storage tank. Her laundry area was also originally situated in the basement.

When her oil furnace died and needed replacement, the service men replaced the aging oil storage tank at the same time. However, they left the old tank in the basement, rather than moving it. They said they would have had to cut the tank up into smaller pieces to haul out of the basement as it had been installed when the house was being built.

It solved their problem, but not my mother's. The original oil tank continued to emit furnace fuel fumes, which triggered respiratory reactions in my mother.

Moving the laundry room onto the main floor helped my mother and she stayed away from the basement area.

Action Item: If practical, move laundry facilities to the first floor.

Is the furniture i.e. living room chairs and couches, kitchen chairs, etc. Easy for the elder to get in and out of?

Rationale: The elder may have difficulty getting in and out of low furniture.

Action Item: Remove small and low furniture.

Large Screen Televisions:

Rationale: With larger screen televisions becoming commonplace, a hazard can be created for an elder who may be unsteady on their feet. A trip or a stumble can cause an unsecured television to fall, creating an electrical and/or glass breakage hazard.

Action Item: Stabilize unsecured large screen televisions to the wall with a security strap. These can be purchased at electronics or hardware stores.

Safety Devices:

Use a Reacher device.

Rationale: Reacher devices are an inexpensive and effective tool for extending the reach of an elder. Yours too for that matter.

Be sure to not lift anything breakable or too heavy when using a Reacher device.

Action Item: Obtain a Reacher device and demonstrate to the elder how to use it.

Floor to ceiling pole:

Rationale: Many elderly have mobility problems making getting in and out of their bed or bathtub, or perhaps their favorite chair, quite difficult for them to manage

There are several inexpensive models of floor to ceiling poles on the market that can be easily installed. Multiple poles can be purchased and installed in key areas such as the elder's bedroom, their bathroom and the living room.

Action Items:

1. Install a floor to ceiling pole or other assistive devices for the person to hold on to when rising from furniture.
2. You should demonstrate to the elder how to use the equipment safely and effectively. They should also be monitored to ensure they follow through with using it appropriately.

[Author's Comments] My mother took on an expanded role as caregiver to my father after he had his right leg amputated above the knee as a result of out-of-control diabetes.

My father was a heavy man. More so after his surgery as he was unable to exercise.

Even after being fitted for an artificial leg, he balked at strength-building exercises as he was terrified of falling. Previous tumbles to the floor had resulted in my mother calling the local ambulance services to pick him up off the floor and set him upright again.

He put psychological pressure on my mother to help him into and out of his bed. This put physical stress on my mother, causing her to experience her own physical problems.

I believe that if floor to ceiling poles like this were available at the time, it would have made life easier for both of my parents. It would have my father take more responsibility for his mobility and would have reduced my mother's aches and pains.

Hip pads:

Action Item: Encourage the elder to wear hip pads should they be at risk for falls.

Seating at the Home Entrance:

Make it Safe TIP: Install a seat at the entrance of your home to remove or put on your shoes and boots.

Safety Suggestions:

Go slow up and down stairs.

Rationale: Don't rush going up or down stairs. Rushing is a major cause of falls.

Eye glasses and climbing stairs:

Does the elder remove their reading glasses when using the stairs?

Keep it Safe TIP: Car keys should be inaccessible. This assumes of course that the elder is no longer driving and/or may be confused.

Firearms should be kept in a gun safe or off the property.

IN THE NEXT CHAPTER WE FOCUS ON ASSESSING FALL HAZARDS IN THE elder's home.

ASSESSING FALL HAZARDS

In this chapter we look at potential fall hazards within the elder's home and offer solutions to prevent them.

Rationale: Falls often cause injuries. Some injuries, such as a broken hip, can be serious. Older people are more likely to break bones in falls because many older people have porous, fragile bones (osteoporosis). Some injuries caused by a fall are fatal.

According to Mr. Google... falls are the leading cause of death from injury among people 65 and older. Approximately 9,500 deaths in older Americans are associated with falls each year. More than half of all fatal falls involve people 75 or over. Among people aged 65 to 69, one out of every 200 falls results in a hip fracture.

Risk factors for falls in the elderly include increasing age, medication use, cognitive impairment and sensory deficits.

FALLS ARE THE LEADING CAUSE OF FATAL AND NON-FATAL INJURIES for older Americans. Falls threaten seniors' safety and independence and generate enormous economic and personal costs.

According to the U.S. Centers for Disease Control and Prevention:

One in four Americans aged 65+ falls each year.

Every 11 seconds, an older adult is treated in the emergency room for a fall; every 19 minutes, an older adult dies from a fall.

Falls are the leading cause of fatal injury and the most common cause of nonfatal trauma-related hospital admissions among older adults.

Source: National Council on Aging - Falls Prevention Facts https://www.ncoa.org/news/resources-for-reporters/get-the-facts/falls-prevention-facts/

Remove Fall Hazards.

To reduce the risk of falls for seniors, one of the most important actions you can take is to make the home fall-safe.

Safety Assessment Question: Do the steps of the stairs have a non-skid surface?

Action Item: Install nonskid treads on steps if not present.

Note: We discuss steps and stairs in depth in upcoming chapters.

Safety Assessment Question: Are there solid handrails on both sides of the stairway?

Action Item: If handrails are not present, install a handrail on at least one side of the stairway.

Safety Assessment Question: Are pets underfoot?

Action Item: This isn't an easy question to supply an action for. Many pets are clingy and tend to stay very close to their owners. If the elder requires the in-house services of a healthcare professional, it might be a good idea to secure the pet in another closed room for the duration of the visit.

Safety Assessment Question: Are household pathways clear?

Considerations: Consider developing storage or organization systems to help deal with the clutter.

Action Items:

1. Ensure household pathways are clear.
2. Remove clutter.

Safety Assessment Question: Does the elder wear anti-slip footwear within the house?

Action Item: Encourage the elder to wear supportive, ant-slip footwear within the house as well as when outdoors.

Safety Assessment Question: Are there grade changes at entrances or between flooring changes?

Action Item: Adjust grade changes at entrances or between flooring changes.

Safety Assessment Question: Do door sills present a potential tripping hazard?

Action Items:

1. If possible, adjust threshold entryways to remove a difference in elevations between rooms.
2. Paint door sills with a different highlighting color to help avoid tripping.

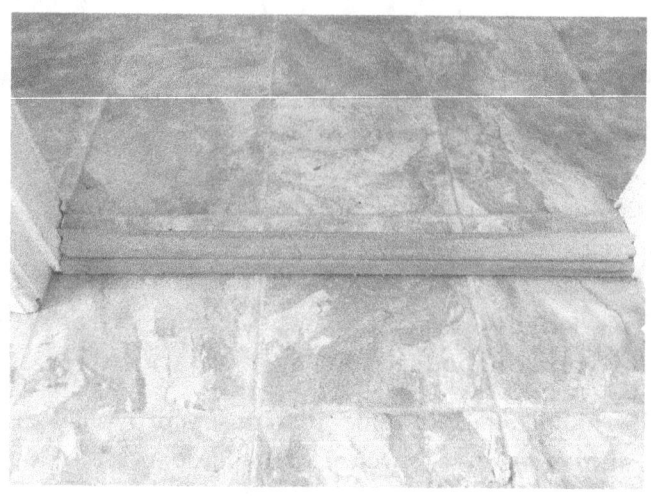

SAFETY ASSESSMENT QUESTION: IS THERE ANY CLUTTER ON the stairs?

Action Item:

1. Ensure there is no clutter or obstacles on the stairs.
2. Clean up loose clutter. This includes newspapers, loose clothing and shoes.

MAKE IT SAFE!

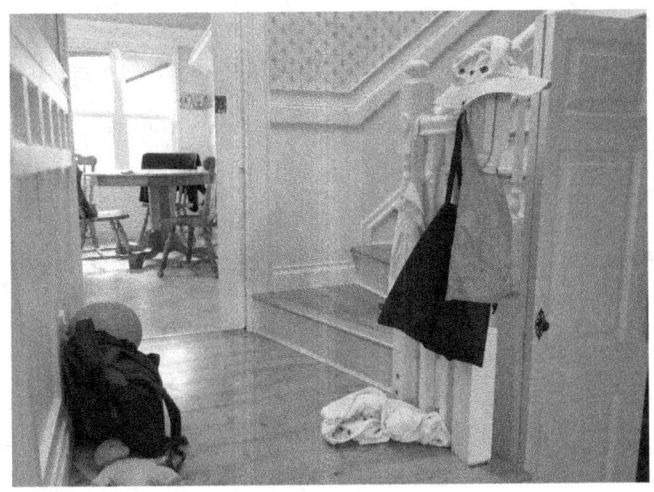

Safety Assessment Question: Is the elder able to climb and descend stairs easily or with difficulty?

Action Item: If stairs are too difficult for older adults to safely use, consider installing a stair glide or having the elder stay on the main level.

Safety Assessment Question: Are there any small furniture items that could be a trip hazard?

Action Items:

1. To prevent fall risks, use cord covers for all cords and cables, or secure them out of the way, behind furniture.
2. If carpet is loose or wrinkled, or the floors are damaged or uneven, have them repaired.
3. Remove foot stools and small tables from the living room if not essential to the elder's functioning.

Safety Assessment Question: Are the home's high-traffic areas clear of obstacles?

Action Item: As you walk through the home, consider how it would be for an elder to navigate with a cane, a walker or a wheelchair.

Considerations: If obstacles to navigation are identified, is it possible to remove the obstacle or change it so that it doesn't provide a hazard?

Safety Assessment Question: If you use floor wax, do you use the non-skid kind?

[Author's Comments] I'm reminded of when I was younger and my mother would wax the hardwood floor in our living room. My brothers and sisters and I would slide around the floor in our sock feet as if we were on a skating rink. Inevitably, somebody would fall and hurt themselves.

This type of floor wax would certainly be hazardous to an elder, especially if they aren't wearing non-lip footwear.

Action Item: If floor wax is required, switch to the non-skid type.

IN THE NEXT CHAPTER WE LOOK AT SAFETY HAZARDS IN SPECIFIC areas of the home, starting with hallways and stairwells.

HOME SAFETY - HALLWAYS & STAIRWELLS

In this chapter we look at safety hazards in specific areas of the home, starting with hallways and stairwells.

SAFETY ASSESSMENT:

Action: Do a walk around safety assessment.

Take the **Home Safety Assessment Form** with you and do a walk about inspection of the hallways and stairwells of the elder's home.

As mentioned earlier, there may be some duplication of the possible hazards identified and solutions offered.

Safety Assessment Question: Are household pathways clear?

Considerations: Consider developing storage or organization systems to help deal with the clutter.

Action Items:

1. Ensure household pathways are clear.

2. Remove clutter.

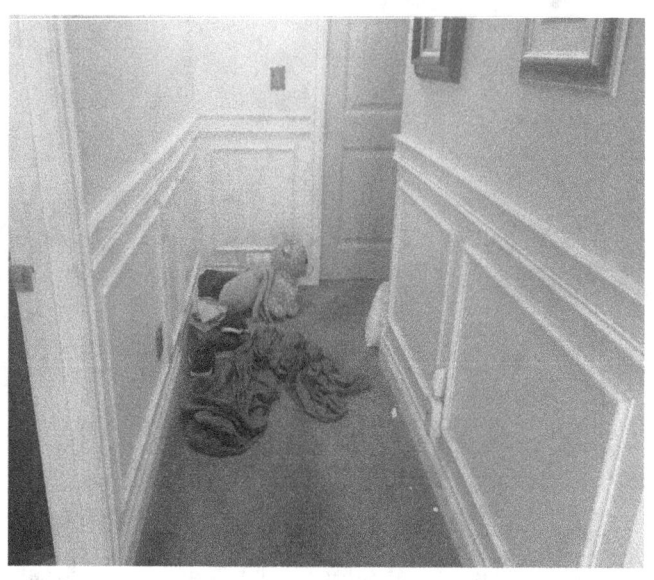

SAFETY ASSESSMENT QUESTION: DO THE STEPS OF YOUR STAIRS have a non-skid surface?

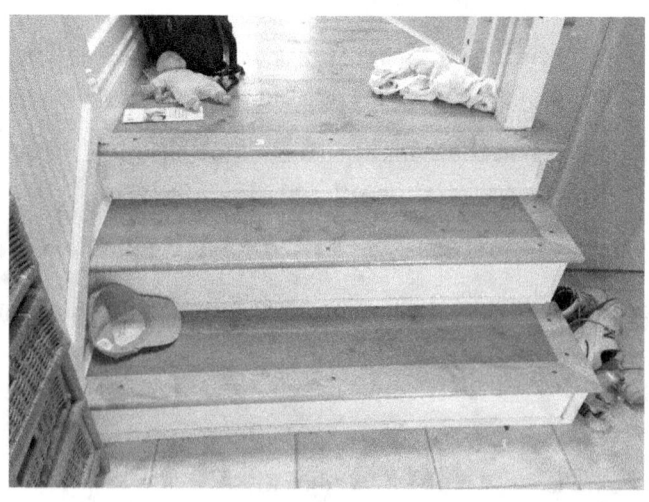

MAKE IT SAFE!

ACTION ITEMS:

1. If stairs are difficult for older adults to safely use, consider installing a stair glide or having the elder stay on the main level.
2. Install rubber stair treads to provide grip to an otherwise slippery set of stairs.

[Author's Comments] I grew up in a tri-story, split-level house, meaning there were three main floors. Five, if you include the two levels of the basement.

The largest staircase was between the living room and the bedrooms level. They were wooden painted stairs, without any treads.

As children, they came in handy for indoor toboggan rides, sliding down the slippery stairs on our pillows. It made for a bumpy ride, but it was a lot of fun.

Not so much fun though when we were going down the steps in our socks and went flying down them when we slipped. It seemed every family member had their own misadventure on these stairs.

We were always amazed and grateful when my aging grandmother visited and managed to leave without a major injury from these stairs.

It took a good twenty years before my parents installed treads on the stairs. They finally installed a hand railing at the same time.

It's amazing nobody was seriously injured in all those years and falls.

Safety Assessment Question: Are there light switches at the top and bottom of staircases and/or hallways?

Rationale: Older homes may only have a light switch installed at the bottom of the staircase or one end of the hallway. This would necessitate you having to go back to the source to turn it off again, which could create risk walking in the dark.

Action Item: Install light switches at the top and bottom of your staircases. This installation would require the services of a qualified electrician.

Safety Assessment Question: Is there adequate lighting for safely moving in the hallway or stairwell?

Rationale: The existing light fixtures may be adequate if a suitable light bulb is installed. There are a variety of lightbulbs available e.g. halogen and LED that provide more light, last longer, shed less heat and are more economical to operate.

Action Item: Ensure there is good lighting in stairways and hallways.

Consideration: If good lighting is not present e.g. inappropriately placed, it may be necessary to contact a qualified electrician to install additional fixtures.

Safety Assessment Question: Is there clutter or obstacles on the stairs?

Rationale: Clothing, books, etc. can easily pile up at the top and bottom of the stairs waiting for someone to carry them up or down at the next opportunity.

With many elderly experiencing visual challenges, these piles of clutter can easily become a trip hazard for them or anyone else for that matter.

Action Item: Ensure there is no clutter or obstacles on the stairs.

Considerations: Some people find it helpful to keep a laundry basket near the stairs, but not so it creates a hazard, to store items to be taken to the next level when enough of a load is gathered.

Safety Assessment Question: Are there solid handrails on both sides of the stairway?

MAKE IT SAFE!

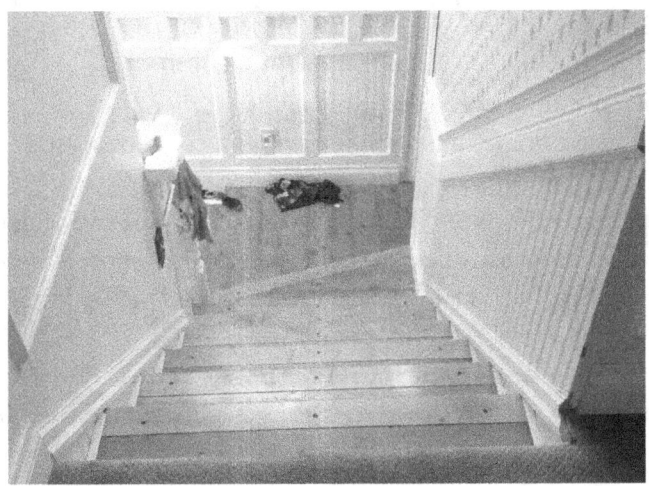

Rationale: You don't have to be a home handyman to do this. Grab the railing and try to shake it back and forth. If the railing wiggles (even somewhat), it's time to fix it. Tighten all nuts and bolts or replace the railing.

Action Items:

1. If stair railings are present, test them for stability.
2. If solid handrails are not present in stairways, install them on both sides of the stairs. If you are handy or have access to a handy person, this is relatively easily done.

Considerations: It's essential the railing holders are securely fastened to the wall's studs. The railings should not cause more of a hazard than they are attempting to solve. An example might be where the rails protrude into the passageway, making it too narrow to navigate safely.

Safety Assessment Question: Is it easy to differentiate one step from another?

Rationale: With partial vision, an elder may be unable to separate one step from the next. This could increase the chance of the elder falling or slipping.

Action Items:

1. Differentiate between stair steps.
2. To increase home safety for seniors, you could paint stair tops a contrasting color.
3. Stretching a piece of different colored duct tape over the top of each stair can also make each step easier to spot. Ensure the tape doesn't become loose and create its own safety hazard.

Safety Assessment Question: Are there grade changes at entrances or between flooring changes that could be a trip hazard?

Rationale: Many elders have visual difficulties which can include depth perception or the inability to differentiate between two surfaces.

Considerations: Wood or metal thresholds are available at building centers. They can be cut to length and can come in various widths to accommodate the grade difference between two areas of the house.

Action Items:

1. Adjust grade changes at entrances or between flooring changes.
2. Paint door sills with a different highlighting color, by serving as a visual cue, can help avoid tripping.

Safety Assessment Question: Does the elder wear anti-slip footwear?

Rationale: Many floor surfaces can be slippery for an elder to walk on. It is often compounded by the elder wearing footwear that might be deemed comfortable rather than safe and practical.

Action Item: Encourage the elder to wear anti-slip slippers or anti-slip socks when walking around your home, especially on slippery surfaces such as polished hardwood floors or tile.

Pool or bathing shoes may be an option for the elder when getting in and out of a bathtub.

Safety Assessment Question: Does the elder remove their reading glasses when using the stairs?

Rationale: Reading glasses are designed for seeing close up. Wearing them while walking up or down stairs may not provide adequate vision to navigate the stairs or to identify hazards.

Action Items:

1. Encourage the elder to remove their reading glasses before navigating stairs.
2. Encourage them to not rush going up or down stairs. Rushing is a major cause of falls.

Considerations: Rushing to answer a telephone can be a cause of falls in the elderly.

Action Item: Provide a portable, cordless phone on each floor of the elder's home to reduce the need to rush to answer a phone.

IN THE NEXT CHAPTER WE LOOK AT POTENTIAL SAFETY HAZARDS IN the kitchen.

HOME SAFETY - KITCHEN

The kitchen is often the heart of a home. Therefore, it seems only fitting that you should spend considerable time making this room safe for an elder.

Do a walk around safety assessment.

Take the **Home Safety Assessment Form** with you and do a walk about inspection of the kitchen of the elder's home.

Go on pantry patrol.

Safety Assessment Question: Does the refrigerator contain outdated or expired food items?

Safety Assessment Question: Food safety: Do food items have proper storage, expiry dates?

Action Item: Check for proper storage of foods. Example: food products requiring refrigeration after the product is opened.

Rationale: You probably won't have any problems if foods not requiring refrigeration are placed in the fridge. However, products such as dairy products that aren't refrigerated would likely be spoiled and should be disposed.

Action Item: Check products for expiry dates and/or best before dates.

Safety Assessment Question: Is a thermometer present and is the fridge within a safe operating temperature?

Rationale: People with dementia may eat spoiled, expired, raw and moldy food.

Action Item: Make regular pantry and refrigerator inspections. Discard any stored foods past their "best before" date.

If necessary, adjust the refrigerator's temperature to ensure it is in the safe operating range.

Make it Safe TIP: [From Mr. Google...] The U.S. Food and Drug Administration (FDA) says the recommended refrigerator temperature is below 40°F; the ideal freezer temp is below 0°F.

However, the ideal refrigerator temperature is actually lower: Aim to stay between 35° and 38°F (or 1.7 to 3.3°C).

[Author's Comments] My mother-in-law lost her sense of smell in the later part of her life. She lived alone, independently, and was not aware of items in her refrigerator that may have spoiled.

When we visited her, it was often evident that something was 'off.'

Your sense of smell can provide you with a clue to investigate further.

Make it Safe TIP: [From Mr. Google...]

Which Foods Can Be Contaminated With Mold?

Mold can grow on almost all foods.

That said, some types of food are more prone to mold growth than others.

Fresh food with a high water content is particularly vulnerable. On the other hand, preservatives decrease the likelihood of mold growth, as well as the growth of microorganisms.

Mold does not only grow in your food at home. It can grow during the food production process too, including throughout growing, harvesting, storage or processing.

Common Foods That Can Grow Mold

Below are a few common foods that mold loves to grow on:

Fruits: Including strawberries, oranges, grapes, apples and raspberries

Vegetables: Including tomatoes, bell peppers, cauliflower and carrots

Bread: Especially when it contains no preservatives

Cheese: Both soft and hard varieties

Mold can also grow on other foods, including meat, nuts, milk and processed food.

Most molds need oxygen to live, which is why they usually don't thrive where oxygen is limited. However, mold can easily grow on food that has been packed in airtight packaging after it has been opened.

Most molds also need moisture to live, but a certain type called xerophilic mold can occasionally grow in dry, sugary environments. Xerophilic molds can sometimes be found on chocolate, dried fruits and baked goods.

Can you eat food with mold on it?

While you probably won't die from eating fungus, keep in mind that foods that are moldy may also have invisible bacteria growing along with the mold. The colorful mold you see on the surface of food is just the tip of what is going on inside.

Most molds are harmless, but some are dangerous. Some contain mycotoxins.

These are poisonous substances produced by certain molds found primarily in grain and nut crops, but are also known to be on celery, grape juice, apples, and other produce. These substances are often

MAKE IT SAFE!

contained in and around the threads that burrow into the food and can cause allergic reactions or respiratory problems.

What to do if you see mold on your food?

Don't eat—throw these out if you see mold:

Luncheon meats, bacon, or hot dogs, cooked leftover meat and poultry, cooked casseroles, cooked grain and pasta, soft cheese (such as cottage, cream cheese, Neufchatel, chevre, Bel Paese) crumbled, shredded, and sliced cheeses (all types), yogurt and sour cream, peanut butter, legumes and nuts, bread and baked goods.

Jams and jellies (The mold could be producing a mycotoxin. Microbiologists recommend against scooping out the mold and using the remaining condiment.)

Cheese made with mold (such as Roquefort, blue, Gorgonzola, Stilton, Brie, Camembert)

Eat—after cutting off the mold

Hard salami and dry-cured country hams (Eat them. Scrub mold from the surface. It is normal for these shelf-stable products to have surface mold.)

Firm fruits and vegetables (such as cabbage, bell peppers, carrots, etc.) as well as hard cheeses are okay to eat if you remove the mold. Cut off at least 1 inch around and below the mold spot. Keep the knife out of the mold itself so it will not cross-contaminate other parts of the produce.

Remember while you're preparing all this food, removing mold, etc. that you should be washing your hands and food prep surfaces often.

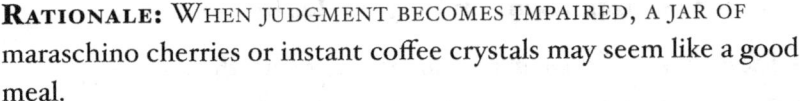

RATIONALE: WHEN JUDGMENT BECOMES IMPAIRED, A JAR OF maraschino cherries or instant coffee crystals may seem like a good meal.

Action Items:

1. Put certain foods out of sight.
2. This might seem odd... but limit your pet's mealtimes and remove the bowl so your loved one doesn't snack on kibble.

Safety Assessment Question: Are commonly used items stored towards the front of the fridge?

Action Item: Store commonly used items towards the front of the fridge.

MAKE IT SAFE TIP: KEEP A CLOSE EYE ON EVERYDAY appliances or permanent fixtures that can become hazards.

Safety Assessment Question: Is there a stable step stool (with a safety rail) for reaching high places?

Action Item: If it is necessary for an elder to reach into upper cupboards, ensure a step stool with a stable base and a handrail is available. It should be within easy reach for the elder. Look for a stool no more than one or two steps in height.

Safety Assessment Question: Is food easy for the elder to find without using stools or ladders?

Rationale: Climbing on step stools, chairs or counters is risky for people with dementia, visual perception problems or balancing problems.

Action Item: Make food easy to find and reach.

Safety Assessment Question: Is the elder able to buy groceries independently? & does the elder keep a well-stocked pantry and a variety of fresh fruit and vegetables on hand?

Considerations: If the elder is independent with their grocery shopping, provide assistance where needed e.g. transporting the elder to the grocery store, carrying groceries into the house from the vehicle, helping to put groceries away in kitchen cupboards or other storage areas.

If the elder is not independent...

Action Items:

1. Consult with the elder to create a shopping list.
2. If practical, take the elder with you grocery shopping.
3. Stock their pantry with healthy snacks (e.g. yogurt, granola bars, nuts, cheese and crackers, and fruit).

Safety Assessment Question: Are heavy items stored in the lower cupboards and light items in the higher cupboards?

Rationale: Minimize both the need to carry items and the distance the items need to be carried.

Action Item: Store heavy items in the lower cupboards and light items in the higher cupboards.

Safety Assessment Question: Are all the items regularly used in the kitchen within reach?

Action Item: Place all items you frequently use within easy reach in the kitchen – don't place them on high shelves that are hard to access.

Safety Assessment Question: Do items need to be carried a distance to the kitchen?

Action Items:

1. If the elder is not able to buy groceries independently suggest using a grocery delivery or a meal delivery service.
2. Minimize both the need to carry items and the distance the items need to be carried.

Safety Assessment Question: Are pots and pans, canned goods

and staple foods stored in an easy-to-reach location--between knee and shoulder heights?

Action Item: Store pots & pans, canned goods and staple foods in an easy-to-reach location... between knee and shoulder height to minimize reaching and lifting heavy items.

Safety Assessment Question: Are spills wiped up immediately?

Action Item: Ensure that spills are wiped up immediately.

Provide paper towels for clean-up.

Cooking:

Safety Assessment Question: Does the elder wear loose clothing when cooking?

Action Item: If the elder does wear loose clothing when cooking, encourage them to change to something more form-fitting as loose fabric can catch fire very quickly.

[Author's Comments] I'm aware of several people who were badly burned as children when they were cooking and their clothing caught on fire.

Make it Safe TIP: All fabrics will burn, but some are more combustible than others.

Untreated natural fibers such as cotton, linen and silk burn more readily than wool, which is more difficult to ignite and burns with a low flame velocity.

The weight and weave of the fabric will affect how easily the material will ignite and burn.

Fabrics with a tight weave - wool, modacrylic, 100 percent polyester and those that are flame-retardant treated are good choices. Heavy, tight weave fabrics will burn more slowly than loose weave, light fabrics of the same material. The surface texture of the fabric also affects flammability. Fabrics with long, loose, fluffy pile or "brushed" nap will ignite more readily than fabrics with a hard, tight surface, and in some cases will result in flames flashing across the fabric surface.

Most synthetic fabrics, such as nylon, acrylic or polyester, resist ignition. However, once ignited, the fabrics melt. This hot, sticky, melted substance causes localized and extremely severe burns. When natural and synthetic fibers are blended, the hazard may increase because the combination of high rate of burning and fabric melting usually will result in serious burns. In some cases, the hazard may be greater than that of either fabric individually.

Source: City of Phoenix - Flammable Fabrics https://www.phoenix.gov/fire/safety-information/home/fabrics

Safety Assessment Question: Are there automatic devices to turn off the stove & oven?

Action Item: Replace an older kettle with an automatic shut-off mechanism.

Safety Assessment Question: Does the elder point pot handles away from the edge of the stove when cooking?

Action Item: Encourage your elder to point pot handles away from the front edge of the stove. This ensures that they won't bump into them or catch the handles with their sleeve.

Safety Assessment Question: Are the stove knobs/dials accessible to the elder?

Action Item: If the elder has difficulty reaching stove knobs, have them use a stove knob turner. Or consider appliances with the knobs at the front of the appliance.

Safety Assessment Question: Are kitchen counters easy for the elder to reach?

Action Item: Check to ensure your kitchen counters are easy for the elder to reach. If they are too high, it's a good idea to lower them to a more accessible height.

Safety Assessment Question: Are oven mitts within easy reach when the elder is cooking?

Action Item: Ensure oven mitts are within easy reach when the elder is cooking.

Make it Safe TIP: Use heat-resistant oven mitts rather than potholders; they provide a better grip on hot containers and give you better protection against splatters and steam. If you do experience a burn, immerse in cool water (not ice or butter!).

Safety Assessment Question: Are knives stored safely?

Action Item: Store knives and electric appliances in a cabinet with a childproof lock.

Safety Assessment Question: Are kitchen work areas adequately illuminated?

Action Item: Make home lighting brighter but prevent glare.

Safety Assessment Question: Are appliance cords in good condition?

Action Item: If any appliance power cords or wires are torn or frayed, replace them immediately to decrease the risk of fire.

Safety Assessment Question: Are hazardous items stored separately from food?

Action Item: Store hazardous items separate from food.

Hazardous items examples:

- Household cleaning products
- Bleach
- Soaps & detergents

Safety Assessment Question: Are the "off" and "on" positions on the stove dials clearly marked?

Action Item: Ensure the on and off stove dials are clearly marked.

Safety Assessment Question: Are there scatter mats or throw rugs in use in the kitchen?

Rationale: These may be decorative but often lack a rubberized backing to better grip the floor, which can become a trip and fall hazard.

Action Items:

1. Remove scatter mats/throw rugs.
2. If carpet is loose or wrinkled or the floors are damaged or uneven, have them repaired.

Safety Assessment Question: Are faucets easy to turn on and off?

Action Item: Provide rubberized water faucet covers for the kitchen sink. These can be easier to grip and turn and are color-coded: red for hot and blue for cold. You should be able to find these products at a senior's supply store.

Alternatively, you could replace standard 'twist and turn' kitchen water faucet handles with 'single-lever' handles instead. Older people can find these far easier to use.

Safety Assessment Question: Does the elder use the stove or oven for supplementary heat?

Action Item: Heat the home safely – do not use an oven as a heating source, under any circumstance. Turn off all portable heaters when leaving the home.

Safety Assessment Question: Does the elder use a grease splash guard when cooking greasy foods?

Action Items:

1. Wipe off any spilled grease from the stove.
2. Use a grease splash guard when cooking bacon or other greasy foods.

3. Consider using a microwave rather than the stove.

Safety Assessment Question: Is the hot water temperature set to prevent scalds?

Action Item: If you have a water heater, don't set the thermostat to 'Hot'. Instead, use the 'Medium' setting to avoid burns or scalding.

Safety Assessment Question: Are smoke & carbon monoxide detectors in place and with charged batteries?

Rationale: Remember that carbon monoxide is a deadly, odorless, colorless gas – you cannot smell it or see it. Having a working carbon monoxide detector is crucial to elder safety!

Action Item: Keep your smoke detectors and carbon monoxide detectors up to date by checking the batteries regularly and promptly replacing expired/discharged batteries.

Note: If your smoke or carbon monoxide detectors are more than 10 years old, it's time to replace them!

Safety Assessment Question: Does the elder have a cordless phone within easy reach?

Action Item: Have a cordless phone at home and keep it within easy reach, to prevent having to rush to answer when the phone rings.

Safety Assessment Question: Are power cords or power bars in use? Are they overloaded?

Action Item: Do not overload power sockets or extension cords.

Safety Assessment Question: Do you have a fire extinguisher in the kitchen, mounted on the wall away from the stove?

Action Items:

1. Is the fire extinguisher regularly checked to see if it is in good operating order?
2. Is there a record of checking available?

Safety Assessment Question: Are emergency numbers posted e.g. Poison Control, family members?

Action Item: Ensure emergency numbers are posted e.g. Poison Control, family members.

Safety Assessment Question: Does the elder use a walking aid?

Considerations: Does the layout of the kitchen allow for the elder to navigate safely around the Kitchen?

Action Item: Ensure the walking aid is set for the correct height for the elder.

Remove obstacles from the kitchen to allow the elder to navigate safely with or without a walking aid.

Safety Assessment Question: Is the elder aware of foods that may interact adversely with their medications?

Considerations: Are others aware of possible adverse reactions? One common food to avoid when taking cardiac medications is grapefruits and/or grapefruit juice.

Closely related to food and medication interactions are allergies.

Action Items:

1. Research the elder's medications to determine if there are any known adverse interactions to food.
2. Interview your elder to learn if they have any allergies you need to be aware of.

Safety Devices for the kitchen:

Automatic stove shut off device:

Considerations: Consider using automatic devices to turn off the stove and oven or installing an induction cooktop -- which turns off when a pot is removed from the burner. Automatic shutoffs on small appliances are recommended.

Action Item: Install an automatic device to turn off the stove after a set period if no movement is detected.

We talk about stove shut off devices in greater depth in our upcoming chapter on <u>Electrical Safety</u>.

IN THE NEXT CHAPTER WE ASSESS SAFETY HAZARDS IN THE ELDER'S bathroom.

HOME SAFETY – BATHROOMS

In this chapter we assess safety hazards in the elder's bathroom.

ACTION ITEM: TAKE THE **HOME SAFETY ASSESSMENT FORM** with you and do a walk about inspection of the bathroom the elder uses on a regular basis.

Safety Assessment Question: Is the bathroom clean and tidy?

Rationale: The condition of the elder's bathroom can often be used as a determination of how the elder is functioning. That is, if the bathroom is clean and tidy, odds are they are doing well in other areas of daily living. Generally, older women tend to be more concerned with cleanliness than older men are.

Safety Assessment Question: Are all electrical outlets in the bathroom GFCIs? Are they tested regularly?

Rationale: A ground fault circuit interrupter (GFCI) will close the circuit should a person with wet hands come in contact with the receptacle, preventing the individual from being electrocuted.

Action Item: Ensure outlets in the bathroom have a ground fault circuit interrupter (GFCI) or are protected by a GFCI circuit.

Safety Assessment Question: If incontinence products are being used, are the used supplies being disposed of properly?

Rationale: Soiled incontinence products can cause unsanitary conditions if left to accumulate.

Action Items:

1. Provide a disposal collection container separate from regular bathroom waste.
2. Dispose of soiled incontinence products as necessary.

Safety Assessment Question: Does the elder's bathroom door lock have an emergency release so it can be unlocked from both sides?

Action Item: Install bathroom door locks that can be easily opened from the outside should an elder accidentally lock themselves in.

Safety Assessment Question: Does the elder use a walking aid?

Action Items:

1. Ensure walking aids are the correct height for the elder.
2. Ensure there is enough room for maneuverability for the elder in the bathroom. This would include allowing for walkers and wheelchairs if in use.

Fall & Slipping Prevention:

Safety Assessment Question: Do bathmats next to the tub or shower have rubberized backing to prevent the elder from slipping?

Action Item: Utilize rubber backed bathmats to prevent the elder from slipping when getting in or out of the shower or bath tub.

Considerations: Having two or three bathmats available can ensure continued slip prevention when one or more mats are being laundered.

Safety Assessment Question: Are grab bars present, properly placed and well anchored to the wall beside the bathtub or in the shower?

Rationale: Many grab bars are designed to also serve as towel bars, toilet paper holders and in-shower shelves.

Action Item: Ensure there are grab bars present for the elder for toileting and bathing i.e. shower and/or tub.

Safety Assessment Question: If an elder prefers or is required to use a shower, are grab bars and a nonslip flooring in place?

Rationale: Shower seats and shower rails make it much easier and safer for a senior to take a shower or bath without falling, and non-slip mats placed in the tub contribute to staying balanced.

Action Items:

1. Ensure grab bars are available within the shower.
2. Ensure the floor to the shower is slip proof. This can be accomplished by using a removable rubber or vinyl bathmat.

There are also adhesive bath treads designed for shower stall floors that can easily be applied.

An additional option is an anti-slip coating that can be applied to bathtub bottoms and shower bases.

Anti-slip coatings will increase friction and reduce the likelihood of a fall. The components include either a clear coat or a color-matched coating with a semi-transparent powder added to provide a textured surface.

Safety Assessment Question: Does the bathtub have a skid

proof bottom? Are grab rails available? is there a bathmat with a non-slip bottom?

Action Item: See Action Items in the above safety assessment question.

Safety Assessment Question: Are there any trip hazards in the bathroom e.g. loose mats?

Action Item: Remove any trip hazards. Examples: throw rugs, stools, etc.

Minimize clutter.

Safety Assessment Question: If it's difficult for the elder to take a shower standing up, have they considered a bath seat?

Action Items:

1. Place a special bathing chair in the tub. Your best choice for a bathing chair is one that will also fit in the shower.
2. Install a hand-held, easily reachable showerhead. These can be easier to use, especially when cleaning hard-to-reach places.

Safety Assessment Question: Does the elder fear getting in and/or out of the bathtub?

Action Items:

1. Encourage the elder to bathe only when help is available.
2. A family member the elder is comfortable with should be designated to be available to assist the elder with bathing.
3. It can be helpful to set up a schedule for bath days.
4. If you are assisting an elder to bathe or supervising their bathing, this can be a good time to observe their physical condition for signs of bruising, malnutrition, dehydration etc.

Safety Assessment Question: Are cold and hot faucets clearly marked?

Action Item: Ensure cold and hot faucets are clearly marked.

Safety Assessment Question: Is the hot water temperature set to the recommended 49°C (120°F) to prevent scalding?

Safety Assessment Question: Is a water temperature regulator present?

Rationale: As we age, our skin becomes more sensitive to temperature changes and we can burn easier.

Action Item: Set the hot water heater to Medium to prevent scalding.

Safety Assessment Question: Does the elder test the water temperature before they get into the bathtub or shower?

Rationale: Many elders prefer warmer water than what we may prefer, so you would need to know their preferences.

Action Item: The elder should be encouraged to test the water temperature before entering.

~

SAFETY ASSESSMENT QUESTION: IS THE ELDER ABLE TO USE the toilet independently and safely?

Considerations: If the elder has difficulty getting on and off the toilet, a raised toilet seat and a well-anchored grab bar can help.

Toilets should be between 17 and 19 inches in height. Seniors will find it easier to sit and stand.

Action Item: Replace the original toilet seat with a raised toilet seat with handlebars.

Safety Assessment Question: Are cold and hot faucets clearly marked?

Safety Assessment Question: Is there a night light in the bathroom?

Action Item: Ensure there is a night light available in the bathroom that automatically turns on in the dark.

Safety Assessment Question: If medication is stored in the bathroom, is it safe & secure?

Action Item: Put medicines in a lockbox and block access to cleaning supplies and razors.

Consideration: You may want to switch to a cordless electric shaver for elderly men.

Safety Assessment Question: Do bathroom cleaning products in use create slipperiness?

Rationale: Some tile and bath cleaning products actually increase slipperiness when applied to flooring. Be careful when using such products.

Action Item: Assess cleaning products used in the bathroom. They should not create a hazard when being used to solve a different problem.

Safety Assessment Question: Are bathroom cleaning products harsh or caustic?

Rationale: Harsh smelling cleaning products can create or add to existing respiratory conditions. They may trigger a breathing crisis. As bathrooms tend to be smaller rooms, especially in older homes, they don't usually provide adequate ventilation for harsh cleaning products.

Action Item: Purchase cleaning products that are safe to use, i.e. nontoxic.

Provide additional ventilation such as opening a window if it is necessary to use a harsh smelling product.

Safety Assessment Question: Is mildew present in the bathroom?

Rationale: We discussed mold related to food products in the chapter on kitchen safety.

According to Mr. Google... mold and mildew are types of fungi; typically, mold is black or green, and mildew is gray or white.

Mold tends to grow on food, whereas mildew is an issue on damp surfaces, like bathroom walls, basement walls, or fabrics. Mold grows in the form of multicellular filaments or hyphae, while mildew has flat growth.

The Risk:

People at high risk for mildew-related health ailments include immuno-compromised patients and those elderly with existing respiratory conditions. Health problems due to mold and mildew likely occur when people inhale large quantities of spores.

Symptoms:

The symptoms and severity of mold exposure will vary depending on many factors, including the concentration of exposure, the type of mold, and the overall health of the individual. However, mold exposure generally involves nasal and sinus congestion, coughing and sore throats, tightness in the chest, and difficulty breathing.

Mold releases spores, which are reproductive organisms that create new colonies. These microscopic spores can be inhaled, creating indoor air quality issues for people with asthma or anyone who has allergies to these substances.

Some indoor molds do more than just produce spores. They can also create dangerous mycotoxins or black mold. These toxins can be absorbed into the body, including the skin, intestines, and airways. When inside the body, the toxins can cause adverse health effects that range from mild irritation to respiratory problems.

Prolonged exposure to mold can create significant issues as well. These issues include hypersensitivity, pulmonary injury, and possibly cancer.

Signs of mold/mildew:

If you suspect mold may be present, there are a few signs that you should watch for, but none is more important than smell. Mold has a distinct earthy, musty smell, much like the smell of rotting wood or leaves. It can give you an indication of mold in the home, and if you discover stronger smells in one part of the house, you may have an idea of where the mold is located.

The next sign of mold will be visibly spotting the mold, but this can be harder to discover than the smell. It might seem obvious, but many people actually don't see some of the mold that has been in the house, either because it is too small or because it is hiding in a corner. They could also see it but mistake it for dirt or soot.

Water problems are not proof of mold growth, but they are a sign that mold could appear in the home. If there has been moisture in the home, it's more likely that mold will be present. Keep an eye out for water stains, puddling, damp carpets, and leaky areas near the foundation. Peeling, bubbling, or cracking of paint or wall paper could also be an indicator that moisture is present in the home and mold could be right around the corner.

Another indicator of mold is leaky pipes. If you have leaky pipes anywhere in the home, your chances of mold growth are significantly higher. Make sure all pipes are properly sealed, and if the plumbing is outdated, you may need to seek professional help to replace the pipes, drains, or seals.

Simple Tips for Removing Mold in an Elder's House

Removing mold is a simple process, but in some cases you may need to hire a professional, particularly if widespread and found in multiple rooms. You'll also need to consider how much time you can dedicate to mold-cleaning. If you can't spend as much time, then perhaps you should hire a professional so you know it will be done quickly and effectively.

If you decide to remove mold yourself, be prepared for some physical work. With the right cleaning materials and a lot of effort, you can remove mold, and one of the best ways to kill mold is by using a bleach solution.

Bleach kills the mold and its spores, making it an effective way to remove the fungus. Simply spray a mixture of bleach and water (roughly 1 part bleach, 10 parts water) onto the mold and use a rag to rub it into the surface. This will kill the mold and remove it from your home. You can also use vinegar, borax, hydrogen peroxide, and many other chemicals to remove mold from the home.

The best technique, however, is prevention. By maintaining a clean, dry home with good ventilation, you will reduce the chances of mold ever becoming a problem.

Source: https://www.oransi.com/page/health-effects-mold-elderly

Mold & Mildew Prevention:

To prevent mildew at home, keep all areas moisture-free.

Bathrooms without an exhaust fan can easily cause a build-up of moisture, especially if showers are taken frequently.

Vinyl shower curtains and shower doors can be a source of mildew development if they don't have adequate ventilation to dry completely between showers.

There are mildew removers available at stores to eliminate mildew.

Action Items: If the bathroom does not have an exhaust fan, it may be advisable to install one. This may require the services of a qualified electrician.

Wiping down a vinyl shower curtain or shower door with a dry towel after a shower can help reduce excess moisture.

Safety Assessment Question: Is the elder able to use the telephone? Is telephone accessible in an emergency?

Action Item: The elder should be encouraged to take a portable cordless phone into the bathroom with them in case of an emergency.

Safety Measures for the Bathroom:

Action Item: If the elder is showing early signs of dementia, there may be value in removing the bathroom mirror. Seeing an unfamiliar face looking back at them may be startling.

Action Items:

1. Install grab bars as needed. Towel racks, soap dishes or toilet paper holders should not be used for support.
2. Ensure there is additional lighting.
3. Install a nightlight in the bathroom. This will help elders who may make repeated trips to the bathroom overnight.
4. Install a nightlight or two on the route to the bathroom as well so elders can find their way.
5. Install a handheld shower head.

Lever handles on faucets are recommended.

Renovations or retrofits:

If you are installing a new bathroom for your family member, consider a frameless walk-in shower with a sloped floor instead of a step-over threshold.

Safety Devices for the Bathroom:

Equipment for bathing: A shower chair or bathtub transfer bench is recommended.

Devices to raise the height of the toilet such as a raised toilet seat or commode over the toilet can make it easier for the elder.

Anti-scalding devices can also be used to ensure an inappropriate temperature of hot water does not injure the bathing elderly person.

Audio Monitors: If an emergency develops in a given room where a senior is alone, wall-mounted speakers provide effective communication with others in the home and alert someone that a potentially dangerous situation has occurred.

GPS watches: Modern technology can help greatly with home safety for seniors who might be bothered by bouts of disorientation and given to wandering.

GPS watches can quickly locate a senior who may have left the premises and gone down the street somewhere. It is not uncommon to find disoriented seniors wandering the streets, many blocks from home.

Home security system: Not to be overlooked in the parade of situational devices, home security systems can be of critical value in establishing a safe environment. Especially in cases where an elder must be left alone for a time, these systems can be invaluable in discouraging or preventing entry (or even wandering). Would-be burglars aware that elders are home alone and tempted to target them could thus be effectively kept from carrying out malicious intentions.

Medical alert system: Medical alert systems are one of the most popular methods of monitoring elder safety at home and ensuring that an elder is not left alone in the event of a health crisis or accident which may have occurred. These systems are generally monitored by emergency medical technicians or certified operators, who understand medical conditions, and are prepared to initiate a fast response so that a crisis can be averted.

[Author's Comments] After my father had passed, my mother lived independently for a while. She had the foresight to purchase a medical alert neck pendant.

On one occasion she was standing on a chair in her kitchen to adjust the curtains. She lost her balance and went tumbling to the floor.

She was uninjured but was unable to get herself into a position to get up and standing. She activated her medical pendant and a couple paramedics came to her rescue.

Her comments to me after her ordeal were "I'm okay with a couple young guys coming to see me... but this wasn't what I had in mind!"

She was grateful for having made the decision to purchase the medical pendant. It is unknown how long she would have been on the floor until she was able to get herself up and about again.

Daily activities of the elder that may increase risk:

The elder should be encouraged to wear anti-slip slippers or socks when walking around the home, especially on slippery surfaces such as polished hardwood floors or tile.

IN THE NEXT CHAPTER WE ASSESS HAZARDS IN THE ELDER'S BEDROOM.

HOME SAFETY – BEDROOMS

Y ou may not think danger can lurk in an elder's bedroom, but think again! Elders can encounter several potential risks here.

Action: Do a walk about assessment

Take the **Home Safety Assessment Form** with you and do a walk about inspection of the elder's bedroom.

Safety Assessment Question: Is there a clear path from the elder's bed to the bathroom?

Considerations: If there isn't a clear path from the elder's bed to the bathroom, is it possible to rearrange the bedroom furniture to improve the route?

Action Item: If necessary, make changes to the elder's route to the bathroom from their bed.

Safety Assessment Question: Is there a phone and a list of emergency phone numbers near the elder's bed?

Action Items:

1. Create a list of emergency & frequently used numbers and place near a phone in the elder's bedroom.
2. Have a portable phone available which would allow the elder to carry it around the home as needed.

Safety Assessment Question: Are there night lights or other sources of light on in case the elder gets up in the middle of the night?

Rationale: Nightlights are inexpensive to purchase. A nightlight should be installed in an area that would illuminate the path to the bathroom should the elder need to visit it during the night.

Nightlights should have automatic on/off sensors.

Action Item: If an electrical outlet is not available along the path, consider purchasing a battery operated one.

Safety Assessment Question: Is there a lamp or a light switch near the elder's bed?

Rationale: Bedroom lamps for the elderly should have a 'touch' on/off feature rather than a push or rotating switch which can be difficult for the elderly to use.

Action Item: Replace bedroom lamps with 'touch' on/off features.

Demonstrate how the new lamps work to the elder.

Safety Assessment Question: Is there a light switch near the entrance to the elder's bedroom?

Safety Measures:

Safety Assessment Question: Is the bed height easy for the elder to get in and out of bed?

Make it Safe TIP: Make sure the elder's bed is not too high or low, so it is easy to get in and out of. You can purchase short bed rails to help the elder steady themselves when getting out of bed.

Action Item: Replace a sagging, softer mattress with a firmer one.

This will be far more comfortable, provide more support, and not trap a resting elder.

Safety Assessment Question: Assess whether door locks are required on bedroom doors to keep the elder out of other rooms or to prevent them from being locked in theirs.

Action Item: Replace a round bedroom doorknob with a single-lever instead. An elder can easily push this lever down to open the door.

Consideration: Consider taking the lock off the elder's door to be certain that no one is locked in or out.

Consideration: You may want to put a lock on your own bedroom door and keep your personal and potentially dangerous items out of the elder's reach.

Safety Devices:

Audio monitor: An audio monitor between the two rooms will let you hear if the elder is out of bed or calling for help.

Action Item: If the elder has mobility challenges, getting in and out of bed can be a problem for them. Fit the bedroom with a telescoping grab bar that extends between the floor and ceiling. This can assist the elder with mobility problems in getting in or out of bed independently.

IN THE NEXT CHAPTER WE ASSESS HAZARDS LOCATED IN THE outdoors surrounding an elder's home.

HOME SAFETY - THE GREAT OUTDOORS

The outdoors isn't necessarily great if it presents a risk for your elder.

If you live in an area that has four distinct seasons, each season can bring its own risk.

Action Item: Take the **Home Safety Assessment Form** with you and do a walk about inspection of the outside of the elder's home.

Safety Assessment Question: Do all entrances have an outdoor light?

Action Item: Ensure pathways and steps have adequate lighting.

Safety Assessment Question: Do the doorways to your balcony or deck have a low sill or threshold?

Action Item: If possible, add a wedge or a new threshold to prevent tripping.

Consideration: Consider painting the repair so the elder can see it better.

Safety Assessment Question: Are there solid handrails on both sides of an outdoor stairway?

As we discussed earlier in our chapter on Home Safety - Hallways & Stairwells...

Action Item: If stair railings <u>are</u> present, test them for stability.

Rationale: You don't have to be a home handyman to do this. Grab the railing and try to shake it back and forth. If the railing wiggles (even somewhat), it's time to fix it. Tighten all nuts and bolts or replace the railing.

Action Item: If solid handrails <u>are not</u> present on outdoor stairways, install them on both sides of the stairs. This may require a skilled tradesperson to install the handrails.

Safety Assessment Question: Do outdoor steps and thresholds cause a hazard for elderly residents?

Action Item: Assess outdoor steps for safety.

Rationale: There are 4 types of hazardous steps—Slippery, Surprise, Short and Irregular.

a) Slippery Step - A slippery step does not have enough grip, especially at the step edge/nosing.

On level surfaces, people generally slip on wet surfaces or from wet shoes.

On stairs or steps, people could slip if there in inadequate support for the ball of the foot.

b) Surprise Step - A surprise step is not clearly visible or expected. It could be at the bottom of a flight or a single unexpected step.

c) Short Step - A short step does not provide adequate support for the ball of the foot for safe forward-facing descent.

d) Irregular Step - An irregular step is longer or shorter than the other steps in a flight.

Source: Health & Safety Authority https://www.hsa.ie/eng/Topics/Slips_Trips_Falls/High-risk_Areas/Stairs_and_Steps/

Safety Assessment Question: Are there stairs outside of the home the elder must navigate to enter/exit the home?

Considerations: If the elder has mobility problems, explore the possibility of installing a mechanical stair lift which can smoothly carry your loved one up or down a flight of stairs.

Alternatively, consider if a wheelchair ramp can be placed at the front side or rear of the home. If land space is limited know that a wheelchair ramp does not have to extend straight out it can be built to a double back on itself or even curled around. Ensure the incline is not too steep and the ramp features secure handrails your parents can pull himself up if need be.

Action Items:

1. Determine if a mechanical stair lift or wheelchair ramp is feasible.
2. Research the costs involved with either initiative.
3. Create a budget if viable.
4. Research to see if any funding is available to offset costs of the renovation.

Safety Assessment Question: Look at access to decks and porch areas. Is there a step to the patio? Is there a sliding door threshold to step over?

Action Item: See previous Assessment question above re steps and thresholds.

Safety Assessment Question: Can the elder reach their mailbox safely and easily?

Action Item: Assess the mailbox for height. If the elder is unable to retrieve their mail due to an inappropriate height for them, adjust as needed.

Safety Assessment Question: Is the number of the house clearly visible from the street and well-lit at night?

Action Item: Ensure the home address is visible during the day or night.

Make it Safe TIP: If you live in a rural area and don't have a visible house number, make sure your name is on your mailbox and keep a clear description of directions to your home (main roads, landmarks, etc.) by each phone in your house.

Make it Safe TIP: Some fire departments provide highly reflective address numbers at low to no cost or they can be purchased on-line.

NEIGHBORHOOD RISKS:

Safety Assessment Question: Are there any risks inherent to the neighborhood of the elder's home?

Action Item: Create a list of possible hazards in the neighborhood that could cause problems for an elder. Example: heavy traffic, busy intersections, schools, shops, etc.

Remain safe in the home:

Action Item: Review common sense safety measures with your elder.

Rationale: It can be tempting to open the door to someone who "looks nice" but beware.

Here are some other **action items** for you to do and to remind them about:

1. Install a peephole in your senior's front door.
2. Do not open the door to strangers when home alone.
3. Place a reminder note on the wall beside the front door saying, "Do you know this person? If not, do not open the door."
4. Always keep windows and doors locked.
5. Install a mail slot in the front door to prevent mail theft.

Safety Assessment Question: Is the home safe for a professional caregiver to visit the home?

Rationale: Professional caregivers are trained to consider their own health and safety first. If the home presents a potential hazard to their personal safety, they may deny service until the hazard has been rectified.

Action Item: Correct or remove any hazards that would prevent a professional care giver from visiting the elder's home.

Safety Assessment Question: Is there patio furniture that would cause problems for an elder to get in and out of?

Considerations: Be cautious of patio furniture as it can be low and difficult for seniors to transfer into or out of.

Action Items:

1. Remove and replace patio furniture that is too low for elders to easily get in and out of.
2. Discard patio furniture that is broken or in need of repair.

Safety Assessment Question: Are there any damaged steps or cracks in outdoor sidewalks?

Considerations: Walking on grass can be difficult for older adults with mobility issues.

Action Items:

1. Check to see if there are paved paths to access gardens or backyards.
2. Secure and repair uneven walkways or patio stones.
3. Repair damaged steps or cracks in outdoor sidewalks.

Safety Assessment Question: Are there any hazards such as leaves and ice on outside pathways?

Action Items:

1. Keep walkways and patios clear of fallen leaves and branches, ice and snow.
2. Corral any toys.
3. Remove hazards such as leaves and ice from outside pathways.

SAFETY ASSESSMENT QUESTION: DOES THE ELDER USE A motorized scooter?

Considerations: If so, do they use it safely?

Have they been trained in its safe use?

Who maintains it?

Safety Assessment Question: Are emergency plans in place such as leaving a key with a neighbor in the case of the elder being locked out?

Action Items:

1. Leave a key with a neighbor you trust, in case the elder is locked out.
2. Remind the elder who has a spare key in case they are locked out.

Safety Assessment Question: Are BBQ grills locked & covered when not in use?

Action Item: Keep the grill locked and covered when not in use.

Safety Assessment Question: If you live in an area that has seasonal snow falls, are there plans in place for timely snow removal?

Rationale: Studies have shown those aged above 55 should not shovel snow. A research team discovered that even with healthy young men, shovelling snow showed a great impact on their physical state – their heart rate and blood pressure increased more than when they exercised on a treadmill.

Combine this with cold air, which causes arteries to constrict and decrease blood supply, and you have a perfect storm for a heart attack.

Source: Country Living https://www.countryliving.com/uk/wellbeing/news/a3030/shovelling-snow-heart-attack-risk/

Action Item: Assuming you are well under 55 years old, capable and available to shovel the elder's driveway and sidewalk, do so.

If not, hire someone to shovel the snow when required.

Miscellaneous Outdoor Safety Devices:

Outdoor motion lights:

Action Item: Install outdoor motion sensor lights and path lights to help the elder see after dark.

Fenced-in yard:

Action Item: A fenced-in yard will allow the elder to go outside. Make sure gates lock.

Pool Safety:

Automatic pool cover:

Action Item: Consider installing an automatic rolling pool cover that is made to withstand the weight of people and locks in place. Use the cover whenever the pool is not monitored by someone capable of rescuing a non-swimmer-- even if you'll just be gone a few minutes.

Pool alarm:

Action Item: Use a pool alarm with an electric sensor that will trip a loud, pulsating alarm -- outside and in the house -- when anyone enters the water. The alarm uses an on-off key.

Pull-up pool ladder:

Action Item: If you have an above-ground pool, a pull-up and locking ladder is a must. Make sure it is properly installed.

Daily activities of the elder that may increase risk:

Safety Assessment Question: Does the elder smoke outside?

Action Items:

1. If so, provide a designated safe and protected from the elements area for the elder to smoke.
2. Fire and wind proof ashtrays should be supplied for outside smoking.
3. Ashtrays should be cleaned and emptied on a regular basis.

In the next chapter we look at safety hazards related to home use medical devices.

HOME USE MEDICAL DEVICES

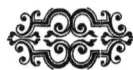

There are many factors that can affect the safe use of medical devices in an elder's home.

A medical device is any product or equipment used to diagnose a disease or other conditions, to cure, to treat or to prevent disease. The Food and Drug Administration's Center for Devices and Radiological Health (USA) regulates medical devices to provide reasonable assurance of their safety and effectiveness.

A home healthcare medical device is any product or equipment used in the home environment by persons who are ill or have disabilities.

These persons, or their providers of care, may need education, training, or other healthcare-related services to use and maintain their devices safely and effectively in their homes or in other places such as work, school, and church.

Examples of some home healthcare devices are ventilators and nebulizers (to help breathing); wheelchairs; infusion pumps; blood glucose meters, apnea monitors, and other home monitoring devices.

Let's start off with the age and structure of the elder's house.

A home's age and structure can affect the quality of care, especially when using medical devices.

For example, older homes may not have the electrical outlets needed for some medical devices. We focus on electrical hazards in an upcoming chapter and expand upon electrical hazards when using electrical medical devices in the home.

Older homes may also have smaller doorways, hallways, and rooms that do not accommodate large medical equipment. Smaller homes may not allow for wheelchairs to pass through the entranceway, forcing patients to use walkers, crutches, or canes instead.

Before a medical device is allowed into the home with an elder, check to see if the medical device is compatible with the elder's home.

Here are some considerations and potential hazards to be aware of.

In-Home Environmental Hazards

Regardless of your geographic location, home settings may present other environmental challenges for the use of medical devices. These challenges include the following:

Pets

Pets may directly interfere with electrical device operation. For example, they may chew through an electrical cord or play with an accessory, such as tubing.

Pets may also contribute to unsanitary conditions where the medical device is used. They may walk over an area that is supposed to be clean, and pet fur/hair may find its way into a device.

Children at Play

Children may interfere with medical device operation. They may change the dial, settings, and on/off switches, twist tubing, adjust machine vents, or remove electrical cords from the outlet. They can also injure themselves while playing with devices they think are toys.

Plumbing

Clean, running water is critical to the use of a medical device in the home. Some medical devices and equipment, such as dialyzers or infusion pumps, require safe water during use, cleaning, and maintenance. Even if water is not required for a device to operate, it may be necessary for cleaning its accessories.

Temperature Extremes

Extreme heat and humidity can negatively affect a working device. Unusually high levels of heat and humidity may:

Cause instruments to operate in unexpected or unusual ways;

Reduce the expected life span of devices or totally destroy products;

Cause laboratory substances used in chemical analysis to lose strength; or

Compromise the cleanliness of packaged devices.

For example, high humidity becomes a problem when a low flow of air causes moisture to build up on a medical device, resulting in a malfunction. Excess moisture may also cause mold to grow on a device.

Dust

Carpets and drapes can hold allergen-containing dust. If dust gets into a medical device, it may affect the way it works.

Fire Hazards

Fire hazards are a concern when considering a home use medical device. Electrical problems with device equipment such as their potential to overheat or short-circuit may increase the likelihood for home fires.

Home care patients who receive supplemental oxygen therapy are also at increased risk. Wherever there is a high concentration of oxygen gas, there is also an increased risk of fire initiated from electrical faults. Taking appropriate fire safety precautions is important.

We will expand upon fire hazards related to oxygen therapy in our chapter on fire safety.

Tripping Hazards

Too much clutter, loose carpeting, and slippery floor surfaces may cause people to fall. Elders who have trouble moving around without the use of a walker, crutch, or cane have a higher risk of falling when these hazards are present.

Poor Lighting

Poor lighting has been shown to result in injuries, especially from falls. Inadequate lighting can also make it more difficult for an elder or caregiver to see and operate a medical device.

Background Noise

There is a lot of noise in the home environment—from vacuum cleaners, televisions, telephones, to people arguing. Outside noise, such as trash pick-up trucks and emergency sirens, is also common. All loud noise can interfere with the ability to hear whether a medical device is operating correctly or whether an alarm has sounded.

Source: Home Healthcare Medical Devices: A Checklist from the U.S. Food & Drug Administration

https://www.fda.gov/medical-devices/home-health-and-consumer-devices/brochure-home-healthcare-medical-devices-checklist

As a homecare medical device user, you should know how your device works.

Action Items:

1. Read your patient education information.
2. Ask your doctor or supplier questions about your device, and take notes.
3. Ask what you need to operate your device.
4. Do you need electricity, running water, telephone, or computer connections to operate your device?

5. Check to see that your home is suited for your device.
6. Do the stairs, doorways, bathrooms, house wiring present any problems?
7. Keep <u>Instructions for Use</u> close to your device.
8. Pay attention to alarms and error messages.
9. Be familiar with what the alarms and error messages mean.
10. Follow Instructions as given.
11. Call supplier for help if you don't understand how your device works.
12. Report to your doctor or device supplier any new problems you have with the device.

Take care of your device and operate it according to the manufacturer's directions.

Action Items:

Read your instructions for taking care of your device and follow them for:

- cleaning
- replacing batteries, filters
- protecting your device (e.g. keep food and drinks away from your device).
- Can you safely take your device from home to school, work, church, and vacation spots?
- Check ahead to see if these other places are suited for your device.
- Dispose of your medical device according to the manufacturer's instructions.
- Always have a back-up plan and supplies.
- Make sure you know what to do if your device fails.
- Have emergency phone numbers for suppliers, homecare agency, doctor, and manufacturer.
- Be sure that you have the after-hour phone numbers.
- If appropriate, keep extra batteries for your device.
- Know how to replace them.

MAKE IT SAFE!

- Educate your family and caregivers about your devices.
- Include them in hospital planning meetings or any device demonstrations.
- Ask them to do a hands-on demonstration to show they can effectively use the device.
- Keep children and pets away from your medical device.
- Don't let children play with dials, settings, on/off switches, tubings, machine vents, or electrical cords.
- Don't allow pets to chew or play with electrical cords.
- Check with your supplier to see if you can turn off your device when not using it.

Contact your doctor and home healthcare team often to review your health condition.

Check to see if there are new conditions that may change the way you or your caregiver use the device.

Are there changes in vision, hearing, ability to move?

Have you had an illness, new medicines, loss of feeling?

Report any serious injuries, deaths, or close calls.

Report these events to FDA at 1-800-332-1088.

Report these events to your supplier.

FDA will take action when needed to protect the public's health.

IN OUR NEXT CHAPTER, WE LOOK AT ELECTRICAL SAFETY HAZARDS and how to avoid them.

ELECTRICAL SAFETY

In this chapter we feature questions, tips and action items related to electrical safety, gathered from the previous chapters for an easy, quick reference and expand upon them where necessary.

If you or your elder live in an older home, it would be wise to have a qualified electrician inspect the house's wiring, fuse box, electrical cords and appliances for safety.

The money you spend on an electrical safety inspection could provide you with some much-needed peace of mind.

Let's start off with assessing the home's lighting.

Rationale: Aging eyes don't always work as they once did. Elders may misjudge or completely avoid darkened areas in their home.

Action Items:

1. Locate and replace any burnt-out light bulbs.
2. Consider substituting the newer lower power consuming and brighter LED bulbs.
3. Test all lighting for effectiveness by standing in one corner of a

room and looking across the room. Can you see a clear path? If not, brighten things up with more lights.
4. Install new light fixtures where needed.
5. Install motion detection lighting inside and outside the home.

Rationale: Motion activated indoor lighting is available in hard-wired and battery operated versions. The battery operated versions can be an ideal solution in areas where installing an electrical fixture isn't practical or is cost prohibitive.

Safety Assessment Question: Is there good lighting in stairways & hallways?

Action Item: Provide effective lighting where required.

Make home lighting brighter but prevent glare.

Safety Assessment Question: Does every room have proper lighting, including walk-in closets?

Action Item: Ensure every room has proper lighting, including walk-in closets. Use a nightlight to make it easy to see at night. Battery operated nightlights are available for areas without electrical access.

Safety Assessment Question: Is there a lamp or a light switch near the elder's bed?

Action Item: Place a light (such as a lamp) close to the bed and make sure the elder can reach it easily.

Bedroom lamps for the elderly should have a 'touch' on/off feature rather than a push or rotating switch which can be difficult for the elderly to use.

Extra lamps-- consider models that turn on and off with a touch of the hand.

Safety Assessment Question: Are there light switches at the top and bottom of your staircases and/or hallways?

Action Item: Install light switches at the top and bottom of your staircases. This installation would require the services of a qualified electrician.

Safety Assessment Question: Is there adequate lighting for safely moving in the hallway or stairwell?

Rationale: The existing light fixtures may be adequate if a suitable light bulb is installed. There are a variety of lightbulbs e.g. halogen and LED that provide more light, last longer, shed less heat and are more economical to operate.

If good lighting is not present e.g. inappropriately placed, it may be necessary to contact a qualified electrician to install additional light fixture(s).

Action Item: Ensure there is good lighting in stairways and hallways.

Safety Assessment Question: Are there night lights or other sources of light in case the elder gets up in the middle of the night?

Rationale: Night-lights are inexpensive to purchase. A nightlight should be installed in an area that would illuminate the path to the bathroom should the elder need to visit it during the night.

If an electrical outlet is not available along the path, consider purchasing a battery operated one.

Night-lights should have automatic on/off sensors.

Action Item: If lighting is not adequate, install new light fixtures along the path between the bathroom and the elder's bedroom.

Safety Assessment Questions: Is there a light switch near the entrance to the elder's bedroom? & Is there a night light in the bathroom?

Action Item: Ensure there is a night light available in the bathroom that automatically comes on in the dark. This will help elders who may make repeated trips to the bathroom overnight.

Ensure that there is additional lighting. Install a nightlight or two on the route to the bathroom as well so that elders can find their way.

Safety Assessment Question: Are controls & switches reachable from a wheelchair or bed?

If possible, are you able to relocate controls and switches so they are reachable from a wheelchair or bed?

Electrical Outlets, power bars & Extension Cords

Safety Assessment Question: Are electrical outlets or powerbars overloaded or used unsafely e.g. daisy-chained?

Rationale: Daisy chaining is where one power bar or extension cord is plugged into another one and possibly even another.

Do not overload power sockets or extension cords.

Action Item: If any of the appliance power cords or wires are torn or frayed, replace them immediately to decrease the risk of fire.

If power cords or extension cords are necessary, purchase ones rated for the energy they are expected to carry and for the correct length.

Make it Safe TIP:

Beware of an acrid burning smell often described as being ozone.

This smell occurs when electrical components have a bad connection and the electricity arcs. It could also be due to electrical burning, and could be the smell of the insulation heating and perhaps melting during a failure.

Whatever the cause, the smell is an indicator you have a potential fire hazard and an appliance or piece of electrical equipment needs to be taken out of service.

If the smell is tracked down to an electrical fixture, a qualified electrician should be called in as soon as possible to fix the problem. Don't use the electrical circuit or appliance until seen by an electrician.

[Author's Comments] For the last decade or so of her life, my mother used an oxygen concentrator on a daily basis. She had emphysema as a result of smoking cigarettes for over thirty years.

An oxygen concentrator is an electrically powered medical device, either by electricity or battery that receives air, purifies it, and then distributes the newly purified air.

She told me that one day she was watching television in her living room and she kept smelling a burnt wiring smell. She was unable to determine where it was coming from.

She stepped into her kitchen for a short moment only to hear a loud explosion sound coming from the living room.

When she went back to the living room, she found a dark cloud of smoke and a stronger electrical smoke smell. Her oxygen concentrator had apparently exploded. The explosion left a layer of black dust on the furniture throughout the living room.

She contacted the supplier, who in turn contacted the manufacturer. They replaced the unit but denied that an explosion of their equipment could happen and it must have been due to user error.

Safety Assessment Question: Are electrical cords or cables exposed in a way that could be a trip hazard?

Action Item: Avoid stretching extension cords across the floor.

Appliance Safety-- Large and Small Appliances

Action Item: Have a professional or plumber clean the vents of your dryer once every three months. Dryer vents cause 2,900 fires every year (USA), and the leading cause of these fires is failure to clean them.

Don't leave your dryer running when you are sleeping, or not at home.

Safety Assessment Question: Are appliance cords in good condition?

Action Item: Service your appliances every 3-6 months.

Rationale: Many seniors keep important medication in their refrigerators, so it's important to make sure they are in good working condition. If you have a clothes dryer, make sure the vents are cleaned by a professional, to prevent risk of fire.

Action Item: If any appliance power cords or wires are torn or frayed, replace them immediately to decrease the risk of fire.

Electrical Safety Devices for the kitchen:

Safety Assessment Question: Is an automatic stove shut off device in place?

Considerations: Consider using automatic devices to turn off the stove and oven or installing an induction cooktop -- which turns off when a pot is removed from the burner.

Automatic shutoffs on small appliances are recommended.

There are 'smart plugs' on the market that allow you to connect any existing stove to the Internet. You can monitor your stove from anywhere, anytime using the Android or Apple app for smartphones and tablets. It requires wireless Internet at the home.

There are also electric stove 'turn-off' products that can increase cooking safety for those with dementia who still have good stove skills and judgment but are liable to forget occasionally. Some of these devices come with a timer, a motion sensor, and an automatic stove shut-off.

Gas stove shut off devices are reported to be in development.

All turn off the stove top and/or the oven, but each one works a little differently. Some features may be safer or more convenient for your needs and/or the person you care for. Here are four things to consider.

Timer. Some units allow you to set how many minutes you want the food to be left cooking unattended and others come with a preset time (eight minutes) that cannot be changed.

Turning Stove Back On. Once the stove has been automatically turned off, some units only require the person to return to the kitchen for the stove to come back on, whereas others must be manually turned off and back on again.

Stove Plug. Some units can only be used with modern, four-prong stove plugs and outlets.

Sensor Placement. Depending on the manufacturer's instructions, the sensor must be placed either to the SIDE of the stove (e.g. under an upper cabinet or on the wall) or ABOVE the stove (e.g., on the range hood, wall, or under the cabinet). The sensor must have an unobstructed view of the user.

Source: The Caring Home https://www.thiscaringhome.org/automatic-stove-turn-off-devices/

Action Item: Install an automatic device to turn off the stove after a set period if no movement is detected.

Electrical Safety Devices for the Bathroom:

Safety Assessment Questions: Are all electrical outlets in the bathroom GFCIs and are they tested regularly?

Action Item: Ensure outlets in the bathroom have a ground fault circuit interrupter (GFCI) or are protected by a GFCI circuit so it will close the circuit should a person with wet hands come in contact with the receptacle.

Home Heating:

Safety Assessment Question: Does the home have an adequate heating system or does the elder use the stove or oven to provide heat?

Action Items:

1. Heat the home safely – do not use an oven as a heating source, under any circumstance.
2. Turn off all portable heaters when you leave your home.

Safety Assessment Question: If the elder uses a space heater,

is it placed well away from flammable substances and materials?

Action Item: Ensure all electrical equipment around the house works properly. This includes air conditioning units – seniors are at higher risk of adverse effects due to high temperatures.

Miscellaneous:

Electric Heating Pads:

Many elders find heating pads to be beneficial in relieving chronic aches and pains.

Any type of heat therapy can help relieve back pain. Yet, heating pads are ideal because they're convenient and portable. They're also electric, so they can be used anywhere in the home, such as lying in bed or sitting on the couch.

Electric heating pads can get hot quickly and injure the skin, so it's important to use them correctly.

Precautions and Safety Tips:

Heating pads are effective for pain management, but they can be dangerous when used improperly. Here are a few safety tips to avoid injury:

- Don't place a heating pad or heated gel pack directly on your skin.
- Wrap it in a towel before applying to skin to avoid burns.
- Don't apply a heating pad to damaged skin.
- Don't fall asleep using a heating pad.
- When using a heating pad, start on the lowest level and slowly increase the heat intensity.

Auto Shutoff Function

Most people, especially elderly persons, are apprehensive about using a heating pad when going to sleep. There is a concern that it may cause burns or irritation. Manufacturers of these innovative products have incorporated an auto-shutoff function that shuts off within two hours. This feature allows you to have a peaceful night's rest.

Temperature Settings

One of the outstanding features of heating pads is the ability to control the temperature. Most models have different heat settings that will allow you to select your preferred level. These may range from four to ten, and thus you can customize your level of comfort. When shopping, you can look out for one with an LED controller for adjusting the heat.

Don't use a heating pad that has a cracked or broken electrical cord.

Electrical Blankets:

Closely related to heating pads, albeit on a larger scale, are electrical blankets.

Many elderly have problems keeping warm and an almost instantly warm blanket can be a problem solver. But they are not without risk.

Here's advice from Nursing Home Help https://nursinghomehelp.org/faq/can-an-electric-blanket-or-heating-pad-be-used-in-a-long-term-care-facility/

Addressing the use of heating pads and electrical blankets from a Medicare and Medicaid certified facilities perspective.

According to the State Operating Manual, "The proper use of electric blankets and heating pads is essential to avoid thermal injuries. These items should not be tucked in or squeezed.

Constriction can cause the internal wires to break. A resident should not go to sleep with an electric blanket or heating pad turned on.

Manufacturer's instructions for use should be followed closely.

Injuries and deaths have been related to burns, and fires related to the use of heating pads. Most deaths are attributable to heating pads that generated fires, but most injuries are burns from prolonged use or inappropriate temperature settings.

Prolonged use on one area of the body can cause a severe burn, even when the heating pad is at a low temperature setting.

The cognitive functioning level or confusion level is probably your best indicator of whether your elder is capable and responsible enough to use an electrical blanket safely or not.

[Author's Comments]

Years ago when I wore a younger man's clothes (credit to Billy Joel) I was a part-time Ambulance Casualty Care Attendant. I recall one instance where we transported an older male to the hospital with what appeared to be second-degree burns. He was bed-bound and a Type One diabetic.

He had fallen asleep with an electrical heating pad covering his lower legs. Diabetics often experience a condition called neuropathy.

Neuropathy is where the outer sheathing (protective covering, also called the myelin sheath) of nerve cells (also called neurons) starts to degenerate.

This is similar to an electrical wire that is covered with insulation, and the insulation is beginning to crumble. Without insulation, the unprotected wire will start short circuiting.

In the same way, when the sheathing of nerve cells degenerate, the signals being transmitted are scrambled, resulting in your body receiving signals that are interpreted as numbness, heat, cold, tingling, pain, etc. in the toes, feet legs, fingers, hands and arms.

In this fellow's instance, it appears when he fell asleep, his legs were actually cooking from the heating pad and his nervous system was not telling him of the hazard.

Electrical Medical Devices:

Home care settings are challenging environments. They are very different from hospitals and often present additional risks to the elderly.

Older homes may not have the electrical outlets needed for some medical devices. Older homes may also have smaller doorways, hallways, and rooms that do not accommodate large medical equipment.

Fire hazards are a concern when considering a home use medical device.

Electrical problems with device equipment such as their potential to overheat or short-circuit may increase the likelihood for home fires.

Home care patients who receive supplemental oxygen therapy are also at increased risk. Wherever there is a high concentration of oxygen gas, there is also an increased risk of fire initiated from electrical faults.

Taking appropriate fire safety precautions is important.

WE LOOK AT FIRE SAFETY AND PREVENTION IN GREATER DEPTH IN the next chapter.

FIRE SAFETY & PREVENTION

We've mentioned fire prevention and safety measures in other chapters as we've moved around the house. This chapter summarizes and expands upon those preventative actions.

SAFETY ASSESSMENT QUESTION: HAVE YOU DEVELOPED AN escape route in case of fire and a fire safety plan?

Rationale: Decreased mobility, sight, hearing or cognitive capabilities may limit a person's ability to take the quick action necessary to escape during a fire emergency. People over the age of 65 are twice as likely to suffer injuries or lose their lives in fires compared to the population-at-large, according to the U.S. Fire Administration, part of the Federal Emergency Management Agency (FEMA).

If you are caring for someone with Alzheimer's or dementia, problems with mobility, or if vision or hearing impaired, there are certain precautions that need to be taken in the event of a house fire. These precautions go above and beyond the traditional fire safety guidelines for all families.

Here are some fire safety tips for elderly people with special needs, provided by the U.S. Fire Administration and the Federal Emergency Management Agency (FEMA):

Mobility impairments

If your elderly loved one uses a cane, walker or wheelchair–or is in a cast due to an injury–traditional escape routes may no longer be viable. One-quarter of victims with physical disabilities were unable to act to save themselves during a fire emergency, according to the U.S Fire Administration.

Check all exits to make sure wheelchairs or walkers can get through the doorways. Make any necessary accommodations (such as installation of exit ramps) to facilitate an emergency escape.

Install flooring material that accommodates artificial limbs or canes.

Keep a phone by the bed for emergency calls in case the person becomes trapped and is unable to escape. Put emergency numbers in the speed dial directory of the phone.

People confined to a wheelchair may want to have a small 'personal use' fire extinguisher mounted in an accessible place on the wheelchair, and become familiar with its use.

When escape is not an option due to impaired mobility, fire protection devices such as sprinkler systems, fire-safe compartment walls, and flame-resistant blankets can be used. The key is to have the room fireproofed before an emergency happens.

Blind/visually impaired

The most important thing a blind or visually impaired person can do to improve his or her chances of surviving a fire is to be prepared ahead of time.

Plan and practice two escape routes from each room in the home. By practicing an escape plan, a blind or visually impaired person can escape to safety, without losing time searching and feeling for an exit.

Committing these actions to memory will serve as an instinctual map to safety.

A blind or visually impaired person will not see the fire, but must rely on other senses—the smell of smoke or the sense of heat emanating from the fire to know where the danger is. Test doors before opening them. Use the back of the hand, reach up high and touch the door, the doorknob, and the space between the door and the frame. If anything feels hot, keep the door shut and use the second exit route.

A person may be forced to crawl along the floor to avoid smoke. It can be very disorienting to crawl when you are used to walking—especially for those who count steps to locate doors and hallways. Place tactile markers along the baseboard of exit routes to help a visually impaired person feel their way to safety.

Hearing impaired

Conventional smoke alarms that sound during a fire aren't effective for someone who is hard of hearing.

Many assistive devices are specially designed to alert hearing-impaired people of an emergency. These include smoke alarms and appliances that use strobe lights and vibration equipment. Vibrating beds and pillows that are wired to a smoke alarm have been developed to awaken people who are deaf or hard of hearing.

Smoke alarms with a strobe light outside the house can catch the attention of neighbors or others who might pass by.

Find out if the 911 or other emergency center is equipped to accept cell phone text messages or text telephone (TTY/TDD) calls.

Alzheimer's or dementia

If your relative has Alzheimer's or dementia, know that even cognitively impaired people oftentimes have an innate understanding that something is wrong during an emergency, and may be more clearheaded than you would imagine.

Remain calm during an emergency. Explain what is happening clearly and simply, but don't expect them to remember specific details. Validate their concerns, but provide clear direction without condescending or losing patience.

Provide a picture book of emergency procedures. A cognitively impaired person may be able to follow visual instructions more easily. Contact your local fire department or the National Fire Protection agency.

Practice escape routes. Cognition tends to improve and worsen at various times for people with Alzheimer's or dementia. If escape is practiced continually, instinct may take over and guide the elder to safety.

The person should sleep in a room that has easy access to the outdoors in case the home needs to be evacuated. A ground floor bedroom is best.

If your parent is in the early stages of dementia and lives alone, alert the fire department ahead of time to their special needs.

Regardless of their disability, all elderly people should live in a home with working smoke alarms and sprinkler systems. A working smoke alarm can reduce the risk of dying in a fire by as much as 60 percent, FEMA says.

Practicing escape plans is also vital for all elders. Knowing their escape plan is one of the most important steps elders can take to save their life in a fire. Plan the escape around your loved one's capabilities. Know at least two exits from every room. Make sure your loved one can unlock all doors and windows.

Source: Aging Care https://www.agingcare.com/articles/fire-safety-for-elderly-148990.htm

Action Items: Give due consideration to the advice offered above and apply it to your situation.

Work with your elder to develop an emergency escape plan that works for them. If the elder lives in your home with you or your family, don't forget to develop an escape route for yourselves.

If the elder's home is in an apartment building are they registered on the apartment building's fire safety plan?

SAFETY ASSESSMENT QUESTION: If the elder uses a portable space heater, is it placed well away from flammable substances and materials?

Safety Assessment Question: If the elder uses a portable space heater, is it plugged into the wall or to an extension cord/power bar?

Rationale: According to Mr. Google... space heaters are behind 79 percent of deadly home heating fires, according to the National Fire Protection Association. Half of those fires start because an object sitting within three feet of the heater got too hot and caught fire, but even plugging the equipment into the wrong outlet could put you in danger.

Cheap power strips shouldn't be used for anything that needs to stay plugged in for long periods of time because they don't have surge protectors. Because they have so much start up energy and because they heat up so quickly and for such a prolonged time, the heat transference goes back down to the power strip and causes it to overheat.

The National Fire Protection Association recommends plugging space heaters directly into the wall and never using an extension cord. But even then, double check that your outlet can handle the energy load. If your space heater requires 20 amps and your outlet is only 15 amps, search for somewhere else to plug it in. To check how many amps yours is, look at the corresponding fuse in the breaker panel, suggests Home Depot.

Source: Readers Digest https://www.rd.com/home/cleaning-organizing/space-heater-fire-risk/

Action Item: Assess whether a portable space heater, if used, is being used safely.

Rationale: Again... from Mr. Google... do not plug any other electrical devices into the same outlet as the heater. Place space heaters on level, flat surfaces. Never place heaters on cabinets, tables, furniture, or carpet, which can overheat and start a fire. Always unplug and safely store the heater when it is not in use.

Considerations: Why is the portable space heater even being used?

Is the home's heating system providing sufficient heat?

Are there cold zones in the house where the elder feels the need to provide additional heat?

If a portable space heater is being used, is it safe?

Is the electrical cord frayed or in good condition?

If a portable space heater is deemed necessary, is this the most appropriate one available?

Does the portable space heater have safety features to prevent fire?

Examples:

Overheat Protection: Room heaters with overheat protection detect when internal components become too hot. When an unsafe temperature is detected, the switch automatically shuts off the unit to prevent overheating.

Tip-Over Protection: A heater equipped with a tip-over protection switch will automatically shut off if it's tipped over for any reason.

Cool-Touch Housing: Cool-touch housing prevents accidental burns by touching the exterior of a heater. This is particularly useful safety feature, particularly in areas with active children or pets.

Action Item: If a portable space heater is in use, provide regular inspection and maintenance.

Occasionally inspect your portable space heater, particularly when you first purchase it. Frequently clean and maintain it to ensure it's working safely.

Wiping yours down will also help reduce the amount of dust and allergens that may be dispersed around your space.

Encourage the elder to unplug the portable space heater when it's not in use.

More Considerations: Keep portable heaters away from water.

Unless it is specifically designed for use in damp spaces, refrain from running a heater in a bathroom or a humid basement. Don't touch the heater if you are wet or have wet hands, as this increases the risk of electrical shock.

PREVENT POISONING: CARBON MONOXIDE

Make it Safe TIP:

- Never try to heat your home with your stove, oven, or grill since these can give off carbon monoxide— a deadly gas that you cannot see or smell.
- Make sure there is a carbon monoxide detector near all bedrooms and be sure to test and replace the battery two times a year.

SAFETY ASSESSMENT QUESTION: IF THE HOME IS OLDER, HAVE you or an electrician inspected the house wiring, fuse box, electrical cords and appliances for safety?

Action Item: Have a professional or plumber clean the vents of your dryer once every three months. Dryer vents cause 2,900 fires every year (USA), and the leading cause of these fires is failure to clean them.

SAFETY ASSESSMENT QUESTION: IF THE ELDER COOKS, DO THEY PRACTICE SAFE COOKING TECHNIQUES?

Hazard: Leaving the stove unattended or cooking at too high heat.

Rationale: One in five Americans admits to leaving food cooking unattended on the stove, found an American Red Cross survey. Walking away from food cooking in the kitchen is a serious fire risk. "The leading cause of home fires is cooking and the leading cause of those fires is unattended cooking."

Hazard: Another potential source of fire is turning the heat too high when cooking.

Cranking up the heat too high can be lethal, even if you're in the kitchen while you cook. Pay close attention and turn off the burner if you see smoke or grease starting to boil while frying food.

Hazard: Having a dirty stove while you cook.

If your stove is covered with grease and other flammable grime, a small kitchen fire can get out of hand quickly. Clean and clear the area around the stove before turning on the heat.

Source: Readers Digest https://www.rd.com/home/improvement/fire-hazards-in-home/

Problems Experienced by many elderly when cooking.

It is known that many older people have difficulties in performing daily living activities such as cooking. These are due to the demands of the tasks and the changes in functional capabilities of the older people...

The findings revealed that the common problems were due to the awkward body position where subjects had to bend down to take things from lower shelves, taking/storing things on higher shelves and cleaning the cooker. Moreover, the safety concerns were the layout of work centres (storage, cooker and sink), the use of cooker and opening packaging. It can be concluded that cooking difficulties are caused by inappropriate kitchen design and the decline of functional capabilities in older people.

Source: Aging: physical difficulties and safety in cooking tasks.

https://www.ncbi.nlm.nih.gov/pubmed/22317518

SAFETY ASSESSMENT QUESTION: DOES YOUR ELDER SMOKE?

Hazard: Not fully extinguishing cigarettes.

While cooking is the leading cause of home fires, smoking is actually the leading cause of home fire deaths. If you have people in your home who smoke, make sure they smoke outside and extinguish all of their cigarettes completely in sand or water.

Source: Readers Digest https://www.rd.com/home/improvement/fire-hazards-in-home/

Considerations: If the elder lives with you in your own home, you can set restrictions where the elder can and cannot smoke.

If the elder lives in their own home you may not be successful in setting smoking restrictions. Long-time smokers can be very set in their ways and can become defensive when limitations are set upon them. Smoking is an addiction and addictive habits have a way of trying to protect the individual from going through withdrawal.

Action Items:

1. The elder should be encouraged to quit smoking for health and safety reasons. At the very least, cutting down on the frequency of smoking can help.
2. The elder should be encouraged to smoke in a designated area, outside.
3. Fire and wind proof ashtrays should be supplied for outside smoking.

4. Ashtrays should be cleaned and emptied on a regular basis.

Safety Assessment Question: Does the elder drink alcohol? Do they drink to excess and increase the potential for hazard? i.e. to themselves or the home?

Considerations: Drinking alcoholic beverages is considered by many people to be one of the perks and pleasures of being an adult. A daily alcoholic drink may be the elder's only pleasure in life. Not my words... but I've heard it many times.

On the other hand, an elder with alcoholism may increase the level of risk.

Action Items:

1. Assess the situation for degree of risk.
2. Develop safety measures to reduce the risk. Examples: only allowing smoking in designated areas outside, etc.

Safety Assessment Question: Are flammable and hazardous materials clearly labeled and properly stored? Is there a designated danger zone in the home to store hazardous chemicals or products?

Rationale: We discussed creating a designated area or danger zone in our previous chapter on Home Safety - Indoors General. The same principles apply to flammable and hazardous materials.

Action Item: Designate a danger zone or remove a hazardous product from the household.

Examples of hazardous products: lighter fluid, barbecue starter fluid, gasoline, portable appliance fuel e.g. butane or propane for hair dryers, kerosene, etc.

GENERAL FIRE PREVENTION SAFETY MEASURES

Change the batteries in smoke and carbon monoxide detectors regularly (after seasonal time changes).

Check the electric cords of all appliances and lamps in your loved one's home. Replace any frayed or damaged cords and limit the number of cords plugged into power strips.

Remove candles from the home. If left burning and unattended, candles can start a fire.

Remind seniors to stay low when exiting the home in a fire. This reduces the chance of smoke inhalation. Coach seniors on how to "stop, drop, and roll" if their clothes ignite.

Discourage the use of portable space heaters. If your loved one insists on using one, place it at least three feet away from curtains, bedding, or furniture. Remind your loved one to turn off the portable space heater before going to bed or leaving the house.

Protect against fires and related hazards

If there is a fire in your home, don't try to put it out. Leave and call 911.

Know at least two ways to get out of your apartment or home.

When you're cooking, don't wear loose clothes or clothes with long sleeves.

Replace appliances that have fraying or damaged electrical cords.

Don't put too many electric cords into one socket or extension cord.

Install a smoke detector and replace the battery twice a year.

Never smoke in bed.

We briefly mentioned hazards related to oxygen therapy in the home back in our chapter on Home Use Medical Devices.

We will expand upon it now.

Oxygen can be both a saviour and a killer. As one of the elements of the fire triangle (heat, fuel and oxygen), it has the potential to kill and injure very easily. However, as a treatment for respiratory and cardiac failure, it is a successful lifesaver.

The enrichment of normal room air with oxygen increases the energy, heat release and severity of any fire. What can normally be a fairly nonflammable substance can, in the presence of oxygen, burn with vigour and produce noxious fumes very rapidly.

Source: https://www.ncbi.nlm.nih.gov/pmc/articles/PMC4487390/

Hazards for home oxygen usage:

Hazard

Specific risks

Tobacco smoking

Burning substances, naked flames (matches, lighters, etc.)

Cooking

Naked gas flames, barbecues (gas or charcoal)

Candles

Birthday cakes, scented candles, decorative candles, lanterns

Household heating

Gas fires, coal fires, log burners, oil fired heaters, etc.

Outdoor

Bonfires, fireworks, gas patio heaters

Flammable materials

Cleaning fluids, paint thinners, petroleum spirit (e.g. for lawn mowers, trimmers and saws), petroleum-based creams or aerosols, alcohols, acetone, some nail-varnish removers, oils, greases or lotions, etc.

Sparks

Grinders, children's toys, some electric shavers

Other

High-frequency, short-wave and laser equipment; hair dryers; arcing, "electronic cigarettes"

The outcomes of fires involving home oxygen use can be categorised into different scales of damage and risk:

- Minor damage to fixtures and fittings.
- Major damage to property (requiring rehousing etc.) and/or minor injury.
- Injury requiring medical treatment.
- Injury requiring hospitalisation.
- Fatality.

The last three categories are more likely to be reported because legislation and reporting systems are usually put in place by oxygen providers, but the size of the home oxygen/house fires and smoking problem is largely under-estimated because smoking patients rarely report minor incidents because they feel they will be blamed for the incident.

Often, visiting healthcare staff or oxygen supply personnel will record indications of smoking damage to property and even burns to the patient. Fires burn hotter and faster in oxygen-enriched atmospheres so usually nonflammable things can ignite at lower temperatures.

The materials that oxygen cannulae are made from, for example, can become highly flammable and cause serious injury irrespective of the poisonous fumes they give off when burning.

Similarly, clothing, bedding and an array of household materials can suddenly become a risk to combustion in the presence of oxygen-enriched air. This is also true for 'electronic cigarettes', which the European Industrial Gases Association has declared to be unsafe to use with home oxygen.

[Author's Comments] On a personal note, my maternal grandmother passed away prematurely due to an oxygen therapy related incident.

My grandmother was a functional alcoholic and a smoker with chronic breathing problems. She was reported to have been having her nightly beer and smoking a cigarette while watching television. Whether she had turned her oxygen off or not is unknown. The theory is she fell asleep and her cigarette either fell onto the couch or her housecoat and ignited.

A passerby noticed the flames in the living room from the street and notified the Fire Department.

My grandmother was taken to the Emergency Department where she passed away due to smoke inhalation.

In an ironic twist of fate, my mother, who lived 100 miles away from my grandmother, was aware of the situation as it was being televised live on the local newscast. She was powerless to do anything about it.

IN OUR NEXT CHAPTER WE LOOK AT CONCERNS ABOUT THE ELDERLY driving and offer some strategies for helping you deal with the challenges involved.

ELDERLY DRIVING CONCERNS

Closely related to assessing safety concerns for the elder you are supporting is the issue of their driving.

It can be an emotionally laden topic for discussion. This chapter explores the issue of elderly drivers from several perspectives and offers helpful strategies to help you resolve your situation.

Aging Drivers Can Present Some Behind-The-Wheel Safety Issues

An aging population with a need for independence can be problematic when it comes to matters related to driving.

Fatality rates for drivers begin to climb after age 65 studies show. From 75 to 84, they are equal to fatality rates of teenage drivers. For drivers 85 and over, the rates are nearly 4 times that of teens. By 2030 all baby boomers will be at least 65 and experts predict they will be responsible for more than a fourth of all fatal crashes.

Source: https://www.roadsafeseniors.org/resources/family-caregiver-resources-and-alternative-transportation/resources-assist-older-road-22

Have you noticed your aging parent is struggling with driving safely? Perhaps there have been a few minor accidents while driving this year. Maybe you have observed a few new dents in their car. For most older adults, losing the ability to drive is cause for serious concern. Most times the elderly driving is proportional to their independence. Taking the car keys away from a senior may cause them to feel depressed or angry if driving is no longer an option.

Often, elderly care issues increase when seniors stop driving. Research indicates that when seniors stop driving, their mental and physical well-being may decline.

However, the consequences of unsafe driving are also significant. According to the Centers for Disease Control and Prevention, more than 6,000 older adults were killed in vehicle accidents in 2015. Further, more than 260,000 older adults were treated in emergency rooms from injuries due to vehicle accidents in the same year.

Suggestions On How To Approach The Elderly Driving Topic:

If you believe it is unsafe for your loved one to continue driving, you are probably dreading talking about it. Here are a few tips you can consider when approaching the subject of senior driving:

Talk to the Doctor: First things first, consult your loved one's geriatrician or primary care physician. The doctor not only knows a detailed medical history but can also provide you with statistics and recommendations for you to use during your conversation. Remember, many older adults have chronic pain or mobility issues that are a danger while driving.

Go in with Empathy: Losing driving ability has a similar feeling to losing the family home for seniors, so go into your conversation with a lot of empathy. This approach can help you to soften your tone while still being firm with your concerns.

Approach and Reproach: The first conversation may have your older loved one on the defensive. If this happens, stop the discussion and return to it another time. You would rather be able to express your concerns and have your loved one listen instead of ending the conversation in an argument or fractured relationship.

Have Specifics: Instead of using general phrases like, "you are not safe to drive," instead use specific examples of times you have been concerned. For example, try saying "You have been in three fender benders in the past six months and it makes me nervous when I know you will be driving." If it helps you to remember your observations, jot them down on a piece of paper before the meeting. This way, you can recall particular accidents or dangerous situations, and their repercussions.

Most Important Is Having Replacement Ideas To Elderly Driving Ready

When you are having the conversation with your loved one, do not forget to provide solutions to their transportation worries. Fortunately, there are plenty of ways and resources that support senior transportation.

Public Transportation: Explore this option of transit in the vicinity. Busses and trains provide accessible transportation throughout town. Many senior specific transportation services are offered through large and more rural areas. Just be aware that these services can only get seniors to and from the desired location. Most times, they do not provide assistance once at the destination. Depending on your loved one's needs and mobility issues, you may find this to be a concern.

Ride Sharing: Another option for transportation includes ride sharing. You may be able to find carpool options for specific activities, like a Bible Study or exercise group.

Uber Health: Read about a new service launched by Uber calledUber Health. They provide transportation on demand or on schedule to assure your loved one can get to and from medical appointments. Typically less expensive than using a taxi, Uber Health is also HIPAA (Health Insurance Portability & Accountability Act - USA) compliant and respects privacy. It allows the ride to be requested by anyone, and riders do not need an account, a phone or to be tech-savvy.

Consider Home Care Services

Finally, if your loved one needs some assistance in getting to a destination, as well as companionship or support during their time there, Home Care services are a great option. A professional caregiver will assist your loved one into the vehicle. Also, they will be with them for the duration of the appointment or trip. This option is excellent for seniors who may have some mobility or cognitive issues, or for a senior who can benefit from some additional companionship and conversation.

If you choose to work with a Home Care agency, assure they do background screening on their caregivers. Also, make sure the agency has insurance on their caregivers while driving the family car. These extra precautions can give you peace of mind and increase the safety of your loved one.

Source: https://hibernianhomecare.com/caregiver/elderly-driving-conversation-loved-one/

A Four-Step Guide To Taking The Keys Away

1. **Identify risk factors prior to becoming an unsafe driver, an older adult may exhibit common signs and risk factors, including:**

- Impaired personal care, such as poor hygiene and grooming
- Impaired ambulation, such as difficulty walking or getting into and out of chairs
- Difficulty with visual tasks
- Impaired attention, memory, language expression, or comprehension
- If you find yourself as a passenger in your loved one's car, you should pay attention to these warning signs. Do they:
- Forget to buckle up
- Disregard signs or traffic lights

- Fail to yield
- Drive too slowly
- Get lost often
- Stop at green lights or at the wrong time
- Fail to notice other cars, walkers, or bike riders on the road
- Veer from the correct lane
- Get honked at or passed often
- React slowly to driving situations
- Mix up the gas or brake pedals, or maneuver them with difficulty
- Drive too cautiously

2. PLAN THE CONVERSATION: IF YOU ARE CONCERNED FOR YOUR loved one's safety and you think that taking the keys away is an appropriate next step, be sure to plan the conversation ahead of time. Don't raise your concerns while your loved one is driving! Wait until they are calm and ready to listen to you.

Often, people who have trouble driving will be very tired afterward. Choose the right time to address the issue with care and compassion. A one-on-one meeting is usually best when talking about sensitive topics. If there are too many people speaking at once, your loved one may feel confused and defensive.

Before having the conversation, research practical solutions. Taking the keys away can seem threatening to your loved one's sense of independence. Come prepared with a plan of transportation options in their area, including home care companies that provide transportation, taxi services, and ride-sharing options, such as Uber or Lyft. Many states have several free public transportation options for seniors.

You may also want to reach out to the local senior center for resources in the area. Offer to accompany your loved one the first few times, so that they feel comfortable. You can also ask your family members, neighbors, and friends if they would be willing to drive your loved one. There are many home-delivery options for groceries and household supplies that can eliminate the need for a trip to a store.

3. Start the Conversation: A good way to start the conversation about taking the keys away is by asking, "How are you doing with driving? Are you still managing or is it becoming difficult for you?" Explain to your loved one that you know this is a difficult discussion. Share your feelings of concern. Listen to your loved one's responses and do not argue. Keep in mind that your loved one is probably worried about losing their independence and becoming isolated from friends and activities. Expect that your loved one may become defensive. Come up with alternative options together and share some of your research. Give specific reasons that explain why you are concerned, including:

A medical condition: A recent diagnosis of cognitive decline warrants consideration if your loved one is still able to drive.

Poor vision: With aging, eyes become more sensitive to light, and night vision becomes more challenging

Recent fender benders or damage to the car.

Getting lost.

Recent tickets or violations.

4. Prepare for Refusal and Next Steps: In an ideal world, your aging loved one will know when it's time to stop driving and the conversation will go well. Unfortunately, most of the time, this delicate conversation about taking the keys away will not end so smoothly. Often the older driver will insist that they are still able to drive.

If the conversation does not go well, do not blame yourself. You can return to this conversation at a later date. Know that you don't need to be the "bad guy." In your next conversation, see if they might be open to having an honest conversation with their physician and taking a driver evaluation test.

Source: https://www.theiaseniorsolutions.com/blog/2019/12/31/taking-the-keys-away-4-step-guide

Five Practical Tips to Keep Your Aging Parent Safe Behind the Wheel

Inevitably, there will come a day when Mom or Dad can no longer drive safely. But if your parent still hasn't reached that point, you'll want to have some strategies in your pocket to help your them stay mobile, independent, and above all, safe.

As the fastest-growing segment of drivers (some estimates suggest that as many as a quarter of all drivers will be over 65 by 2025), it's something most families will have to deal with. So, it's best to be aware of the physical and cognitive changes as well as medical conditions that make driving riskier with age.

And while research shows that seniors tend to have safer driving habits than many of their younger counterparts (they're more likely to wear their seatbelts, and less likely to drive drunk, for example), a 2014 study found that distracted driving may be more dangerous for drivers over 65 due to age-related cognitive decline.

Inevitably, there will come a day when Mom or Dad can no longer drive safely. But if your parent still hasn't reached that point, you'll want to have some strategies in your pocket to help your them stay mobile, independent, and above all, safe.

Here are some ways to help you do just that:

1. Make Sure Your Parent is Healthy Enough to Drive

First thing's first. Make sure your aging loved one is in good shape to drive, both physically and cognitively. A doctor can evaluate him or her to help gauge their ability to drive safely. Some health considerations that frequently affect seniors include vision and hearing problems, so you'll want to ensure your parent has both their hearing and vision tested. Talk to them and their doctors if you're concerned about their ability to hear or see while driving.

Most folks over 65 are taking some type of medication. The question is whether any of those medicines create side effects that could make them drowsy or less alert. If the answer is yes, they'll need to consider limiting or stopping driving.

2. Encourage Exercise

It turns out that exercise has yet another benefit - it can help older adults stay fit to drive. Research has shown that higher levels of physical fitness correlate to better driving performance for senior drivers. That doesn't mean your aging parent needs to sign up for a gym membership or start running marathons. Any physical activity that boosts flexibility should also help improve posture and stave off fatigue while driving. The AAA Foundation for Traffic Safety has created some simple stretching exercises to help seniors improve their flexibility.

3. Check Their Car

Almost as important to senior driving safety as physical fitness is the vehicles seniors are driving. Today's car manufacturers offer a range of features that can help keep older drivers comfortable and safe. Take a look at your parent's vehicle and how they interact with it the next time you see them. Is it easy for them to get in and out of the driver's seat? Once seated, do they have enough legroom, and are they easily able to adjust mirrors and seats?

There are a number of additional features that can address common senior health issues - for example, six-way adjustable seats allow drivers with hip pain to easily adjust their seats in different directions. And a senior with vision problems may benefit from features such as extendable sun visors, larger control buttons, or an auto-dimming rearview mirror.

4. Consider Driver Refresher Courses

Many organizations offer driver refresher courses designed for seniors. While it may take a little convincing to get your aging parent to head back to a physical classroom, there are plenty of on-line classes that can help them re-sharpen their driving skills. And in case they need added incentive, let your parent know that taking one of these classes may actually save them money on car insurance.

5. Limit Driving

If your parent is having trouble driving, limiting where and when he or she drives can help them stay on the road while lowering some risks they face. Some obvious ways to do this would be to avoid driving at night or in bad weather - conditions that can be hazardous for drivers at any age. It's also a good idea for them to refrain from driving at rush hour or to take less-busy roads when possible.

Talking to your aging parent about their driving isn't easy, but having that conversation far outweighs the potential catastrophe that awaits if you ignore the issue. Be sensitive when discussing the subject and make sure your parent knows you'll be there for them when the time comes for them to hand over the keys.

Bottom line - if you think there may be a problem, there probably is. Your aging loved one may drive just fine on surface streets, but so could your 12- year-old. And if something does happen, if they do hurt another person, you could be liable for the damage. Or the death.

Source: https://www.huffpost.com/entry/5-practical-tips-to-keep-_b_9692968

Video: Driver Safety for Older Adults: What Families Need to Know

UCLA's Longevity Center held a community meeting on January 16, 2014 to discuss Driver Safety for Older Adults.

https://www.youtube.com/watch?time_continue=5366&v=xzh5uH_QTiM&feature=emb_logo

Video: Senior Driving https://www.youtube.com/watch?time_continue=26&v=ahKN6AZlucU&feature=emb_logo

Additional Resources:

10 suggestions on how to approach your aging parents driving:

https://www.roadsafeseniors.org/blog/10-suggestions-how-approach-your-aging-parent%E2%80%99s-driving

How to talk to an elderly parent about driving:

https://www.care.com/c/stories/5586/how-to-talk-to-a-parent-about-driving/

4 tips to convince an elderly parent to stop driving:

http://sixtyandme.com/4-tips-to-convince-an-elderly-parent-to-stop-driving/

Seniors and Driving: A Guide

https://www.caring.com/caregivers/senior-driving/

Resources to assist an older road user:

Family/caregiver resources and alternative transportation:

https://www.roadsafeseniors.org/resources/family-caregiver-resources-and-alternative-transportation

Older Drivers video: https://www.youtube.com/watch?time_continue=150&v=-A6gXoZDsXc&feature=emb_logo

IN OUR NEXT CHAPTER WE LOOK AT WHAT YOU NEED TO DO AFTER you've completed your home safety assessment and what you should be looking for on subsequent visits to the elder's home.

ONGOING FOLLOW-UP

In this chapter we explore what you should be looking for on subsequent visits to the elder's home.

Check in with them frequently.

Home safety for elders means checking in with them regularly.

Do you live in the same town or city as the elder you are supporting? Drop in unannounced to get a better idea of how they are truthfully doing. If you don't live close to the elder, arrange with someone else to take on the responsibility of ongoing follow-up.

Considerations: By now you have probably realized how much time and effort is involved in supporting an elder living semi-independently in the community. It can be a little easier, in some ways, when the elder is living in your home with you.

For those elders living semi-independent there may be value in arranging for a maid/cleaning service to visit the elder's home once a week for light housekeeping duties. This would include dusting, vacuuming and cleaning untidy areas of the home. Kitchens and bathrooms often require extra attention.

Several times a year, perhaps quarterly, a deeper cleaning could be organized to include cleaning the windows, vacuuming areas that wouldn't have been done in the regular cleaning e.g. overhead ceiling fan's blades, behind furniture, walls and ceilings, etc.

This, in turn, can take a lot of pressure off you.

Action Items:

1. Be on the lookout for anything that has changed or needs repaired since your last visit.
2. Ask the elder if there is anything broken or needing fixing.
3. Check the kitchen stove/cooktop grease filters to see if they need cleaning.
4. Check on the home's indoor temperature. Is it appropriate compared to outdoor temperatures. Examples: warm in the winter and cooler in the summer if hot outdoors.
5. Is the elder wearing clothing appropriate for the weather conditions?
6. Monitor an elder in extreme hot or cold weather (when the risk of heat stroke or frostbite is higher).
7. Advise the elder to call you for help before trying to tackle a cleaning or repair job independently.
8. While visiting make a list of areas that need tidying and create a list of cleaning supplies that may need to be purchased. If you have the time, clean the area. If not, schedule a time to return and complete the cleaning.
9. Check portable phones for its charge. Replace a low charge phone with a fully charged one from the phone charger.
10. Remind an elder to move more slowly from one room to the next – there is often no reason to rush.
11. Keep a close eye on permanent fixtures that can become hazards -- including garbage disposals, ovens, stove tops and gas fireplaces.
12. Ensure emergency contact phone numbers remain posted in a central location such as the elder's refrigerator.

13. Check refrigerator for signs of food spoilage and expiry dates on food containers.
14. If the elder is a smoker, look for signs of burns on furniture and clothing from cigarettes.
15. Observe the elder for any visible signs of cuts or bruising, which could be indicative of the elder tripping or falling.
16. Observe the elder's home for signs of clutter build up or new hazards that may have developed.
17. If you are supporting an elder who is living semi-independently, set up a regular shopping day with them.
18. Help them develop a shopping list in advance. [Many caregivers find this to be a frustrating task, as the elder tends to want to shop for something when they think of it, not waiting until the designated shopping day.
19. This can result in frequent requests of the caregiver to take the elder shopping which can impinge upon the caregiver's ability to manage their own time.]
20. Stock their pantry with healthy snacks (e.g. yogurt, granola bars, nuts, cheese and crackers, and fruit).

IN OUR NEXT SECTION, SECTION THREE, WE LOOK AT MAINTAINING your elder's ongoing health and welfare with the first chapter focusing on day-to-day healthcare supervision.

SECTION THREE: MAINTAINING THE ELDER'S HEALTH & WELLBEING

DAY TO DAY HEALTHCARE SUPERVISION

Depending on the level of functioning of the elder you are supporting, you many need to advocate on their behalf when interacting with healthcare professionals.

AS MANY ELDERS AGE, THEIR LEVEL OF UNDERSTANDING OF complicated matters, such as we see in healthcare can increase. We shouldn't generalize, though as many elders remain very bright as they age.

WITH OUR ELDER POPULATION REQUIRING INCREASED SUPPORT FROM the healthcare profession as they age, more healthcare practitioners are getting used to interacting with a family member acting as an advocate on behalf of an elder.

THIS SECTION FOCUSES ON TACTICS AND STRATEGIES YOU CAN USE when communicating with healthcare workers on behalf of an elder you are supporting.

How to talk to the Pros

One of the challenges often faced with the elderly in working with their physicians, is they hold the physicians in very high regard. Where a younger person may challenge a physician, or ask for a second opinion, many elders view a physician's word as the word of God. Meaning they would never question it. Many elders are too timid or reluctant to question a doctor or to ask for a better explanation of a health matter, fearing looking stupid.

Over the years this lack of communication between elders and their physicians has added to problems with polypharmacy. If the elder is a poor historian, or the physician doesn't have access to an up-to-date medication profile, complications can occur.

Polypharmacy occurs where the elder may be going to more than one pharmacy to have their medication prescriptions filled. This can result in medications that interact with others the elder is already taking. Certain medications can cause drowsiness, conversely... insomnia. It is not unheard of to have two medications with different names, prescribed by two different doctors for the same problem.

Doctors Visit Plan of Action

If this is the first time you will be advocating on behalf of the elder you are supporting at a doctor's office visit, here are some steps for you to consider:

Prepare for Appointments: When making an appointment, tell the receptionist what the problem is, or the purpose of the appointment, so enough time can be scheduled. Advise the receptionist you will be accompanying the elder to the appointment.

WITH MANY DOCTOR'S OFFICES STARTING TO USE ON-LINE appointment scheduling, you may or may not be able to provide the purpose of your visit.

Set Goals: What do you want to accomplish at this visit?

Know the elder's family history.

Think of what to say. Anticipate questions the doctor is likely to ask. Ask yourself:

• How is the elder affected by this problem?

• What symptoms does the elder have?

• Have they changed?

• How long have they had them?

• How long do they last?

• What do you think caused the problem?

• Is the elder allergic to some medicines?

If it's helpful, make a note of these points.

REMEMBER--THE ELDER IS THE ONLY ONE WHO KNOWS HOW THEY feel.

Write down their symptoms, concerns, and questions before seeing the doctor. Be able to report what drugs, vitamins, and nutritional supplements they are taking.

Note: It is important to remember that you are there to support the elder. If the elder is able to do so, they should take the lead with talking to the doctor. Your support role may be to provide additional details the elder has missed or forgotten. In some cases, you will need to take the lead however, the goal is to help the elder remain independent as long as possible.

Be on time for your appointment.

Don't be shy! Be detailed and specific when describing the elder's problems. Answer the doctor's questions as best you can.

Ask questions. Keep your remarks to the point. Think about what you really want to say.

Focus on one point at a time. Share your needs and concerns. Your doctor is trained to serve as a resource for any health concerns or questions.

Ask if you don't fully understand what the doctor says about:

- How long is the course of treatment?
- Are there any alternatives?
- Are there any side effects to this treatment?
- Where could you go to get a second opinion?
- Are there any tests ordered and why they are needed?
- How the treatment works.
- What the elder must do, including any changes to diet and habits.
- Whether the elder needs to come back and when.

If there's anything else worrying you, mention it before you leave. Make sure you fully understand what the elder needs to do.

DON'T AUTOMATICALLY EXPECT A PRESCRIPTION, BUT IF THE DOCTOR gives you one, be prepared to ask:

- What will it do?
- Does the elder have to take it all?
- When should it be taken? With food? After food?
- Can the elder drink alcohol during this treatment?
- Are there any side effects?
- Raise any issues that the doctor may not know about.

NOTE: It's important to remember to stick with the purpose of the doctor's visit and not introduce multiple problems. Doctors can be very busy, and their receptionists have the challenge of keeping them to schedule, allowing for more patients to be seen.

This is also not the time to bring up your health concerns. Make a separate appointment for yourself.

EXPRESS YOUR HEALTH CONCERNS ABOUT YOUR ELDER.

Think about what you really want to say. If time allows and it is important to you, talk about your rights, beliefs, interests and desires.

In a non-confronting way, state your preferences or why you disagree with what your physician has recommended. (You may want to think about the information and compare notes with a patient advocate before you voice a dissenting opinion.)

Use "I" statements. "I feel this way..." "I would prefer to..." "I understand that you said... is that correct?"

TAKE PART IN THE ELDER'S HEALTHCARE: Get a full explanation of their treatments, the risks involved, expected outcomes, and alternatives. Ask the doctor to explain them again, if you do not understand. Make an informed decision about your treatment. Educate yourself. Ask for reading material.

SEEK YOUR DOCTOR'S ADVICE AS NEEDED: You should have reasonable access to the elder's doctor and his or her staff. Consult with the doctor as the elder's condition dictates and as the doctor's schedule permits.

Confidence and trust between you and your doctor are essential. Look for another doctor if you are having a hard time communicating or do not feel comfortable.

Do not worry about protecting your doctor's feelings. Doctors and patients may have different styles, which are not compatible. Be straightforward and let your doctor know if you are planning on transferring the elder's care to another doctor. This way, all the elder's health records can be transferred to the new provider.

It is very important to talk with your doctor and other health care providers about the needs of the elder you are supporting. Some things you may want to discuss with your doctor include:

- What condition or problem brought the elder to the doctor?

- Questions about medication:

  - What are the side effects?
  - Should the elder take the medication with food?
  - How long will he/she need to take it?
  - What should I look for to see if it is working?

- Questions about the equipment the elder is using:

  - How long will he need to use the equipment?
  - How do I know if it is fitting properly?
  - How do I go about getting equipment?
  - Who do I call when there is something wrong with the equipment?

- Questions about an elder's surgery:

  - When is it, and how long will the procedure take?
  - What will you do during the surgery?
  - How long will the elder be in the hospital or will they go home the same day?
  - What after care is involved? Who will provide it?
  - What are the risks?

- How do we go about getting a second opinion?
- What types of things will the elder be able to do after the surgery?

Follow the rules. Respect the doctor's time by arriving for appointments on time or a few minutes early. If you're unavoidably late, let the office know, and give at least 24 hours' notice for a cancellation or rescheduling.

Follow up. Before you leave the doctor's office, make sure you understand what follow-up appointments or lab tests or blood work the elder needs. Take notes about any instructions so you don't forget them, and if you don't understand how to administer a prescription, ask the nurse or doctor before leaving the office. Communicate with the office, too, if the medication prescribed isn't working or the elder develops worsening or additional symptoms.

THE FOUR "R'S" OF DOCTOR'S VISITS

PATIENTS SHOULD LEARN THE FOUR "R'S" OF DOCTOR'S VISITS... NOT Reading, wRiting and aRithmetic, but key steps to slowing things down and conversing clearly with their doctor.

WRITE: ARRIVE WITH NOTES: THE ELDER'S CURRENT prescriptions, key symptoms and concerns. But don't stop writing at the doctor's office. If you didn't bring a notepad and pen, ask for them.

You'll want to write down medical terms, symptoms and details about recommended treatment. A doctor's visit can be stressful, so even if you listen carefully, details can be lost as soon as you walk out the door. If your doctor is speaking too quickly for you to get down the key points, don't be ashamed to ask for a pause, repetition, or even for help to write it all down.

. . .

REQUEST: REQUESTING CLARIFICATION OF WHAT THE DOCTOR HAS told you can draw out new information by suggesting to the doctor that you want to know as much as you can.

Questions today may also make future visits more efficient for both of you.

SOME EXAMPLES INCLUDE:

- Could you spell that? Spelling a word accurately helps you recognize the word the next time you hear it. It also draws your doctor's attention to the fact that this is a new word to you.
- What does that mean? Now that you know how to spell it, ask for a definition "in plain English"-- and write that down, too. If the definition has more medical terminology, ask again.
- What exactly does my prescription say? Unless you can read the little notations on the slip of paper, you will not know how to check that the pharmacist is supplying you with the correct drug or dosage.

REVIEW: REPEAT WHAT YOU THINK YOU'VE HEARD BACK TO YOUR doctor to check your understanding of the issue and to become more comfortable with new terms. Try using the physician's language and ask if you understand correctly.

This review shows the doctor how comfortable (or not) you are using medical terminology and promotes the use of language you can understand.

Once you get home, review your notes. Do they still make sense to you? If you are confused about something urgent, call the doctor for clarification. If, however, your questions can wait, make sure to write them down and save your notes for the next appointment.

. . .

RELAX: EVEN IN THIS DAY OF SOPHISTICATED SPECIALTIES, COMPLEX treatments and new discoveries, you still need to feel comfortable around your doctors.

Your primary care physician, especially, should work with you to understand your medical condition. You don't need to feel embarrassed about your lack of knowledge, your doctors don't need to feel challenged by your questions.

IN OUR NEXT CHAPTER WE FOCUS ON MEDICATION MANAGEMENT AND safety for the elder's in our care.

MEDICATION MANAGEMENT & SAFETY

Note: The content for this chapter is derived from several different videos available for viewing on-line. The source of the video is cited after each portion of content.

Video: How to Help Your Senior Manage Medication

CARE.COM REPORTED THAT A RECENT STUDY FOUND THAT MORE than 80% of adults aged 57 and older take at least one prescription drug a day. And about half of them regularly mix drugs with over-the-counter medication and supplements. They go on to note that 1 in 25 older adults experience a major drug interaction. Modern medicine has and continues to give us drugs to ease our pain, cure our ills and extend our lives. Advances seem to happen every day and as a result we are seeing more ads on TV, in newspapers and on-line touting the benefits of some new drug.

This is all terrific, but as our parents age and the number of their potential health problems increase, it may mean their doctors prescribe them more and more medicines. Plus, with the holistic health movement, many seniors are using non-medical supplements to improve their overall health.

Because of the volume of medicines and supplements they may be taking, many seniors find they have problems with keeping their medication regimen straight. They may take too much, too little, take it at the wrong time of day or not at all.

What all this means for us the family caregiver is that we have to be extra diligent about helping our senior loved ones manage their medications.

Source: https://www.youtube.com/watch?v=FUlBoM1uh0g&t=2s

VIDEO: SENIOR MEDICATION CHALLENGES: HOW TO HELP Your Senior Manage Medication

Medication Challenges:

According to a survey released in December 2009 by Medco Health Solutions, more than half of the seniors surveyed said they take at least five different prescription drugs regularly and about 25% said they took between 10 and 19 pills each day.

The challenge of managing multiple medications is clear. Nearly 3 in 5 of those surveyed admitted that they forgot to take their medication. Furthermore, the more drugs they used, the more likely they did not remember to take them.

Among those using five or more medications, 53% said they forgot doses, compared to 51% of people who took less medication.

Remembering to take their medication is one problem, but another task that is often a challenge for seniors is getting their medications filled on time.

If your parent is taking multiple medications, or who has frequent changes in prescription or dosages, it can lead to confusion and may cause them to miss taking certain medications.

Getting refills can also be a challenge if your parent is hard of hearing. If his or her pharmacy uses automatic voice prompts, it may be difficult for them to understand, so they might just avoid calling altogether. Getting timely refills can also be a problem if your senior loved one no longer drives.

Many seniors don't want to be a burden to their family and friends, so they may not ask for help to run an errand to the pharmacy in order to get their refills.

Three other medication challenges are:

- Adverse effects

- Side effects

- Drug interactions

EACH OF THESE TERMS HAS A DIFFERENT MEANING.

An *adverse effect* is a harmful or unwanted result caused by medication. Some adverse effects are temporary and only occur when starting, increasing or discontinuing a treatment.

Examples of adverse effects include nausea, constipation or sleepiness.

The problem with adverse effects is if your senior decides the symptom is too troublesome, they may stop taking their medication regimen altogether. Which could result in another, more serious medical problem.

A *side effect* is an unintended result of a medication. Some side-effects can be beneficial such as weight loss, but normally when doctors talk about side-effects, they usually mean adverse effects.

Drug interactions means that medication may interact adversely to another medication, food or beverage. Alcohol is commonly listed as an item to avoid while taking certain medications. But other items such as dairy products and even grapefruit juice can cause harmful interactions.

In all cases you should carefully read the material that comes with each and every prescription to help your parents avoid interaction and understand what is a normal or expected side effect.

Another challenge seniors face is a fear of asking questions. Many don't want to appear silly or uneducated. So instead of asking the doctor or pharmacist for clarification or enquiring if a reaction is normal or not, they just stay silent.

Not having these conversations could result in higher risk of treatment failure or more serious adverse effects.

The high costs of medications can lead to two additional challenges. First, is not taking the medications at the required dose or at all, because they are deemed too expensive. Again, this can lead to treatment failure.

The second challenge is to that to avoid costs, many insurance companies require doctors to order the generic brand of the drug. While generics are often equivalent at a much lower cost, the chemistry of the drug may not have the same effect as the regular brand and your parent may not get the same medicinal benefit they once had.

Other medications may include chewing, non-chewable. Some medications should never be chewed or crushed. Doing so may change how they are absorbed in the body.

Some medications shouldn't be cut because they are coated to be long acting or to protect the stomach. You should also ensure that if your parent has a liquid medication that they use the cup or spoon that came with it in order to avoid dosing errors.

Source: https://www.youtube.com/watch?v=R4jqhnUTWvA

Video: Useful Tips for Managing Medication: How to Help Your Senior Manage Medication

Here are some tips to help your elder manage their medication:

Create a list of all the medications they are taking. Each parent should have their own list. At the top, write their full name and date of birth. List each drug and its dosage.

We also recommend listing any directions. These can be how many times a day and when the medication should be taken, and what foods or liquids should be taken with the medications. Be sure to avoid any food or beverages that should be avoided, such as dairy or alcohol.

This part of the list should also include refill frequency. This list of drugs should include prescriptions as well as any over-the-counter medications and supplements, such as calcium, vitamins and herbs.

Next on the list should be all allergies to medicines and foods.

The last item on the list should be pharmacy and healthcare provider names, address, phone number and family emergency phone numbers.

This list should be readily available for emergency responders. It would be wise to leave a copy on your parent's refrigerator.

Your elder should take it with them to any medical appointment or when filling a new prescription. One or two family members should also have copies and be responsible for updates as necessary.

One of the medication challenges faced by seniors is getting timely refills. If you notice that your parent has prescriptions from multiple pharmacies, work with them to consolidate them to one pharmacy.

You could manage their prescriptions through your e-mail or on-line.

You can share a list of over-the-counter medications with the pharmacist to ensure they won't have any interaction with the medication being taken when combined with a prescription.

When your parent gets a new prescription, be sure to save the materials that came along with it. If you or your parent notices a new issue, such as a memory problem, you can check the reference material to see if a new medication might be causing the problem. This may also be a good time to remind them not to cut or chew tablets unless the directions specifically indicate that it is okay to do.

Perhaps one of the most helpful tools you can offer your parent when managing their medication is an effective organizing system. One of the most common methods is to use a daily pill organizer.

These handy plastic pill organizers can be found at most pharmacies and come in a variety of shapes and sizes. The most common ones usually have seven compartments. One for each day's medication. Others though, have more compartments for each day, so your senior loved one knows what pills to take in the morning, at lunch, dinner or before bedtime.

If you senior loved one has problems remembering to take their medication, there are electronic pill dispensers that will sound an alarm when it's time to take their medication. Other electronic pill reminders talk, relaying information verbally, which can also be very helpful.

No matter what kind of pill organizer your senior loved one uses, you can help by sitting down with them once a week and filling up each compartment for them.

The list you made of all the medications and supplements can serve as a handy reference guide for accomplishing this task. Whether your parent uses a pill organizer or not, it is important they keep the balance of all their medicines in the original containers. The label contains important information such as dosage and expiration date.

It is a good idea for you to check labels for expiration dates on their pill bottles. This is a way for you to help make sure they are getting proper refills and you check the expiration dates and discard any old medication.

Having an open discussion with your parent about their medication and encouraging them to do the same with their healthcare provider and pharmacist is always advisable.

In the end, by speaking up and talking about proper dosages, refills and effects, means your senior loved one's health and quality of life can improve.

. . .

MAKE IT SAFE TIP:

Keep all medications in their original containers so you don't mix up medicines.

Ask your pharmacist to put large-print labels on your medications to make them easier to read.

Take your medications in a well-lit room, so you can see the labels.

Bring all of your pill bottles with you to your healthcare provider's appointments so he or she can look at them and make sure you are taking them correctly.

Source: https://www.youtube.com/watch?v=wxJ3dz8CCLw&t=25s

IN OUR NEXT CHAPTER WE EXPLORE EMERGENCY PREPAREDNESS. Emergencies do happen. Will you be prepared?

EMERGENCY PREPAREDNESS

When you agree to take on the care and responsibility of an elder, whether they live independently in the community and you check on them a couple times a week, or they live semi-independently in your own home and you see them daily, you are taking on an immense amount of commitment and responsibility.

Emergencies involving your elder can tend to happen at inopportune times. An urgent hospital visit or an admission can be stressful for all family members involved, let alone the elder.

This chapter addresses issues of emergency preparedness and offers some solutions to help your peace of mind.

Quick and Easy Access

Planning for quality care does little good if you don't have 24-hour accessibility to your elderly loved ones or having made provisions to access their personal property when an unexpected situation creates the need.

Imagine how you would react if you were unable to reach your elders because you didn't have the key to his or her home. Worse yet, what if you meant to give a set of house keys to your elder's neighbour but you never got around to it and then a neighbour heard your elder's cries for help and could do nothing? Have you given any thought to who would call an ambulance if you were unreachable and an eldercare emergency arises?

• In an emergency, minutes count, getting help could make the difference between life and death.

• The best way to deal with an emergency is to be prepared.

One of the greatest fears of the elderly is one of being alone and hurt when no one else knows.

Keep important telephone numbers handy.

Ensure emergency numbers are posted e.g. poison control, family members. Keep a copy of the emergency information at home and at work.

Post the list near the telephone or on the refrigerator at your home and your elder's home. Keep a copy in your wallet or purse. Update names and phone numbers as needed.

Create check-in systems.

Ideally, your elder will be able to use the telephone to call for help when an emergency occurs. However, this is often not the case. Make a plan for someone to be in contact with your aging family members on a regular basis--by phone, in person, through beepers and e-mail.

Create a network of people who have agreed to stay in touch with your elder.

Consider the protection of a medical alert system.

Identification of hidden medical conditions saves lives in an emergency. Simple options like printed wallet-sized cards and identification bracelets and necklaces are adequate.

Keep vital information accessible.

Store information in one safe, accessible place – at home and/or at work. Updated as needed:

- Emergency telephone numbers
- Blood type
- Medical history
- Medications
- Healthcare number
- Power of attorney
- Driver's license
- Allergies
- Proof of insurance

∾

OUR FINAL CHAPTER LOOKS AT SCAMS TARGETING THE ELDERLY.

SCAMS TARGETING THE ELDERLY

Action Item: Alert your loved one about ongoing scams targeting seniors.

MANY SCAMS ARE UNIVERSAL, FROM THE IRS IMPOSTER WHO CALLS and threatens to arrest you if you don't pay your taxes, to phishing emails that trick you into sending sensitive data or downloading malware onto your computer. **But some types of fraud target older adults specifically or affect them disproportionately**. Older adults may fall for certain scams because they are in the habit of answering calls from unknown callers, open junk mail rather than tossing it in the trash, or are not as practiced with the privacy settings on social media as younger generations.

Here are six scams that you and your parents should watch out for.

Source: Kiplinger https://www.kiplinger.com/slideshow/retirement/T048-S002-6-scams-that-prey-on-the-elderly/index.html?utm_source=SYN-yahoo&utm_medium=referral&rid=SYN-yahoo

Sweepstakes or Lottery: You hear by phone, mail or on-line that you have won—or have the potential to win—a jackpot. But you need to pay a fee, or cover taxes and customs duties, to receive your prize, perhaps by prepaid debit card, wire transfer, money order or cash. Or, the scammer may send you a bogus check that you need to deposit before sending a portion back. **Even if the contest carries a legitimate name, stay away from schemes that require you to pay to claim your prize.** This was the third-most-reported scam in 2018, according to calls received by the Senate Aging Committee's Fraud Hotline (IRS impersonation and robocalls took the top two spots).

1. **Tech Support:** A so-called tech support representative calls and claims that your computer is infected with a virus. Once you hand over remote access, they dig into your personal files or request payment for their services. **Seek tech support only from the contact information provided with your devices.** In 2018, people age 60 and older were about five times more likely to report losing money to these scams than were younger people, with a median loss of $500, according to the Federal Trade Commission.
2. **"Grandchild" in Need:** Your "grandchild" calls—perhaps in the middle of the night, startling you awake—sounding frantic, because he needs fast cash to deal with a medical emergency, a travel disaster or to get out of jail. He begs you not to alert his parents. The con artist on the other end of the line may have extracted enough details about your grandchild from the Internet, such as his or her name, city and school, to weave together a believable story, and may explain away a distorted voice by claiming a bad phone connection or broken nose.

Hang up and call your grandchild or an in-the-know relative to check in.

1. **Romance:** You get a message on an on-line dating site or through social media that says something like "Don't you remember me? I'm your second-grade crush. You look so good!" The seducer may spend weeks or months building a

relationship over phone and e-mail, then **ask for money--perhaps to help him or her travel to you or to deal with medical issues**. These are some of the most devastating victimizations. Some victims can lose hundreds of thousands of dollars--and the dream a scammer created for them.

2. **Social Security:** Someone claiming to be a Social Security staffer contacts you and tries to extract money or personal details. He or she may pretend there is a problem with your account, that your Social Security number has been suspended because of suspected illegal activity, or that you're owed a cost-of-living benefit increase. Worse, **the caller may threaten your benefits, suggest you'll face legal action if you don't provide information, or pressure you to send money**. If you're not sure whether a call is legitimate, don't rely on your caller ID; hang up and call 800-772-1213 to speak with a real representative.

3. **Natural Disasters and Contractors:** Fake contractors will go door-to-door offering fix-it services, often capitalizing on a recent natural disaster in the area. They will ask for instant payment via cash or check, promise to start working the next day, and then disappear. Ignore their offers and **search for contractors on your own**.

WHY ARE THE ELDERLY FREQUENT TARGETS OF FRAUD SCAMS?

Most victims who become the targets of fraud scams are considered to be in the naive segments of the population. Unfortunately, elderly individuals are the most frequent targets of fraud scams. Fraudsters target the elderly, as they may be lonely, willing to listen and are more trusting than younger individuals. Many fraud schemes against the elderly are performed over the telephone, door-to-door or through advertisements. The elderly are prime targets to schemes attributed to credit cards, sweepstakes or contests, charities, health products, magazines, home improvements, equity skimming, investments, banking or wire transfers, and insurance.

What tactics do fraudsters use to take advantage of the elderly?

Fraudsters use different tactics to get the elderly to fall victim to their schemes. They can be friendly, sympathetic and willing to help in some cases or use fear tactics in others. The tactic used is generally dependent upon the type of situation the fraudster finds himself in with the elderly person. For example, a fraudster might focus on home ownership. The fraudster will recommend a "friend" that can perform necessary home repairs at a reasonable price. This friend may require the individual to sign a document upon completion confirming that the repairs have been completed. In some cases, the elderly victim later learns that he signed the title of his house over to the repairman. In other cases, not only is the person overcharged for the work, but the work is not performed properly.

Here are some more common scams targeting seniors?

According to the National Council on Aging (NCOA), the top 10 scams targeting seniors include the following:

1. Medicare-- In scams involving Medicare, fraudsters pose as Medicare representatives to get seniors to give them their personal information, such as their Medicare identification number. The fraudster uses this information to bill Medicare for fraudulent services and then pockets the money.

2. Counterfeit prescription drugs-- As prices for prescription drugs increase, seniors look to the Internet to find cheaper prices for their medications. Unfortunately, fraudsters are aware of this and set up websites that advertise cheap prescription drugs which are usually counterfeit. Seniors who unknowingly purchase these counterfeit drugs soon realize they have been duped when the drugs do not provide any relief from their medical condition or even cause additional health problems.

3. Funerals -- In one type of funeral scheme, fraudsters use obituaries to find out information about the deceased in attempts to extort money from family members or grieving spouses. They claim the deceased has an outstanding debt that must be paid immediately. Those close to the deceased are usually in a vulnerable state and are more likely to pay the fraudulent debt. In another scheme, dishonest funeral directors might try to deceive the elderly by capitalizing on their unfamiliarity of funeral costs and sell them unnecessary services, such as a casket when the deceased is going to be cremated.

4. Anti-aging products-- With society putting so much emphasis on physical appearance, many individuals feel the need to find treatments or products that claim to help them conceal their age. Scammers advertise anti-aging products that are either worthless or harmful. Some products might contain materials that can be harmful, yet touted by scammers as being as effective as a brand name product, such as Botox. Scammers might also advertise products as being effective and natural, but in reality the product has no anti-aging effects.

5. Telephones-- Phone scams are the most common scams used against the elderly. Scammers might get seniors to wire or send them money by claiming to be a family member who is in trouble and needs money. They might also solicit money from the elderly by posing as a fake charity, especially after a natural disaster.

6. Internet-- Since the elderly are usually not as savvy with handling emails and surfing the Internet, they are easy targets for scammers. Victims have been tricked into downloading fake anti-virus software that allows scammers access to personal information on their computers. Seniors might also respond to phishing emails sent by scammers asking them to update their bank or credit card information on a phony website.

7. Investments-- Many seniors plan for retirement or manage their savings after they finish working, which makes them more vulnerable to become victims of investment schemes. Fraudsters can take advantage of victims by posing as financial advisors to get access to their retirement funds and savings. Once they have access to the funds, they take their money and run.

8. Mortgages-- Elderly victims who own their homes can be valuable assets to a scammer. Scammers might send out fraudulent, yet official-looking, letters to victims that list the supposed assessed value of their home. For a fee, the scammers inform them that the value of their home can be reassessed. Scammers might also approach victims about providing home repairs and pressure them to take out equity to use as payment for the repairs.

Source: Association of Certified Fraud Examiners https://www.acfe.com/fraud-examiner.aspx?id=4294997223

Senior Fraud Prevention

Seniors are available because they tend to be retired, they're home, they answer their phones and read their mail. So, some of the offers that come in aren't necessarily more attractive to seniors, but they have the time to read it.

There's still the prevailing idea that seniors grew up in a more polite time when they thought it was rude to hang up on someone and there is the issue of being alone or lonely, so they're more likely to talk to strangers.

According to the NCPC (National Crime Prevention Center), seniors age 60 and over are targets of 49% of telemarketing scams involving medical care services and products, 41% involving sweepstakes and prizes, and 40% involving magazine sales. The NCPC estimates that each victim of a sweepstakes scheme lost an average of $7,000.

PHONE FRAUD

Fraudulent telemarketers use five basic techniques:

Scarcity: The senior has been identified as the grand prizewinner, but if she doesn't accept the prize immediately (and pay that "handling charge") the runner-up will get the prize instead.

Hype: The telemarketer screams and hollers about how excited he is the senior has won.

Authority: The telemarketer passes the phone to his "boss," so his target will know the offer is "legitimate."

Phantom Fixation: The prize is too good to pass up, and the targeted senior becomes fixated on it.

Reciprocity: The telemarketer explains that she won't receive her commission unless the senior accepts the prize and pays the handling fee. When the senior protests that he doesn't have enough money to pay the fee, the scammer asks how much he can afford, and says she'll accept that smaller amount, just because she's so happy the senior has won the prize.

The NCPC has put together a short guide on senior fraud prevention. The guide features five ways to make unwanted telemarketers go away. Tape it by your loved one's phone and he or she will always have a polite-but firm-comeback for unscrupulous come-ons. (Of course, the best way to get rid of someone you don't want to talk to is to simply hang up.)

Tip #1: NEVER GIVE PERSONAL INFORMATION, SUCH AS BANK account or social security numbers, to anyone over the phone, unless you initiated the call and know you've reached the right agency.

Comeback: "I don't give out personal information over the phone. I'll contact the company directly."

Tip #2: Don't believe it if the caller tells you to send money to cover the "handling charge" or to pay taxes.

Comeback: "I shouldn't have to pay for something that's free."

Tip #3: "Limited time offers" shouldn't require you to make a decision on the spot.

Comeback: "I'll think about it and call you back. What's your number?"

Tip #4: Be suspicious of anyone who tells you not to discuss the offer with someone else.

MAKE IT SAFE!

Comeback: "I'll discuss it with my family and friends and get back to you."

Tip #5: If you don't understand all the verbal details, ask for it in writing.

Comeback: "I can't make a decision until I receive written information."

The scammer will most likely keep trying to convince his intended victim, so it's best to hang up after delivering the comeback line.

Practice these comebacks with your loved one. Also, have your loved one tell telemarketers to take his or her name off their call list. If the telemarketers don't, they're breaking the law. Sign up for the National Do Not Call Registry. As a last resort, get your loved one an unlisted phone number.

Fraudulent telemarketers may also use a senior's forgetfulness against them. The scammer may tell her target she's with a well-known charity, and the senior has forgotten to send a check for a pledge.

Most telemarketers can tell when they've got an older person by the voice or inflection of the voice and they will take advantage of it.

Source: A Place For Mom https://www.aplaceformom.com/planning-and-advice/articles/senior-fraud-prevention

CONCLUSION

Congratulations for making it to the end of the book.

I would expect you have discovered many more potential hazards you hadn't considered when you started the home assessment process.

Creating this book and the original Elder Safety session in the Elder@Home Program has been an eye-opener for me as well.

While working in healthcare I found I had a different degree of control over my environment. If I noticed a hazard, I was in a position to either fix it myself or report it and have somebody else responsible for maintenance resolve the problem. Sometimes, it didn't always get fixed as fast as I would have liked.

It's not quite the same at home. It can be easy to get complacent when you're looking at something you see every day that could develop into a hazard. Procrastination can set in with the attitude of "I'll fix that someday."

Many of the pictures I have used throughout the book are of my own home. I hadn't recognized the hazards created when I originally renovated my home.

CONCLUSION

At 65 years of age when writing this book, I consider myself a senior rather than an elder. The clock is ticking as it is for everyone and my elder days are approaching.

Now that I am retired, I have the time to make those household safety improvements as "someday" has arrived for me.

I'm hoping to live in this home for another 10 or 15 years. The safety improvements I make will go a long way in allowing that to happen.

Now the big question is, what are you going to do about it?

If you have read the book, start to finish, without completing the assessment for the elder's home, now's the time to do it.

This can be a daunting task. We covered a lot of different areas throughout the book.

I'm reminded of an old adage that goes "how do you eat an elephant?"

Answer... not that I would ever even consider eating an elephant, the answer is "one bite at a time."

Applying that principle, you may want to focus on one area of the home at a time for your assessment. This will allow you to focus on any hazards you identified and create an action plan you can realistically follow through with. As mentioned in the book, not every problem or hazard can be resolved easily or quickly.

Solving a problem may require a budget. Finding the money for the fix can be a challenge. Will you pay for it out of your pocket or can you have the elder reimburse you for your expenses? This process can take time.

Getting back to the concept of one bite at a time, once you have completed your assessment of a specific area, move on to another area of the home with your assessment.

Don't forget there is a home inspection checklist you can download at https://BookHip.com/SXGMBT and take it with you when you do your home inspection.

CONCLUSION

As an alternative, you may want to consider purchasing the workbook I have created to accompany this book... **Make it Safe! A Family Caregivers Home Safety Assessment for Supporting Elders@Home - Companion Workbook**. The workbook takes the home inspection content from this book and strips it down to the basic Action Items, Considerations and Rationale behind potential hazards in each area of the home.

Each hazardous item identified will also have blank lines included so you may fill in your comments, anything you want to remember or make note of completing your assessment. This workbook is meant to work for you.

In conclusion, I would like to thank you for your interest in your caring to support an elder. As I mentioned in the beginning of the book, it takes a family to support an elder to live as independently as they can, for as long as they can.

ABOUT THE AUTHOR

Rae A. Stonehouse is a Canadian born author & speaker.

His professional career as a Registered Nurse working predominantly in psychiatry/mental health, has spanned four decades.

Rae has embraced the principal of CANI (Constant and Never-ending Improvement) as promoted by thought leaders such as Tony Robbins and brings that philosophy to each of his publications and presentations.

Rae has dedicated the latter segment of his journey through life to overcoming his personal inhibitions.

As a 25+ year member of Toastmasters International he has systematically built his self-confidence and communicating ability.

He is passionate about sharing his lessons with his readers and listeners.

His publications thus far are of the personal/professional development, self-help, self-improvement genre and systematically offer valuable sage advice on specific topics.

His writing style can be described as being conversational. As an author Rae strives to have a one-to-one conversation with each of his readers, very much like having your own personal self-development coach.

Rae is known for having a wry sense of humour that features in his publications. To learn more about Rae A. Stonehouse, visit The Wonderful World of Rae Stonehouse at https://raestonehouse.com

ALSO BY THE AUTHOR

PROtect Yourself! Empowering Tips & Techniques for Personal Safety: A Practical Violence Prevention Manual for Healthcare Workers https://books2read.com/protectyourself

∼

Power of Promotion: On-line Marketing for Toastmasters Club Growth

https://books2read.com/powerofpromotion

∼

You're Hired! Job Search Strategies That Work (This is the complete program)

E-book & Paperback: https://yourehirednow.com

On-line E-course: (Available as a self-directed or instructor-led program) https://liveforexcellenceacademy.com/

∼

You're Hired! Resume Tactics: Job Search Strategies That Work

E-book & Paperback: https://resumetactics.online

On-line E-course: https://liveforexcellenceacademy.com/

∼

Job Interview Preparation: Job Search Strategies That Work

E-book & Paperback: https://jobinterviewpreparation.online/

On-line E-course: https://liveforexcellenceacademy.com/

You're Hired! Leveraging Your Network: Job Search Strategies That Work

E-book & Paperback: https://leveragingyournetwork.online/

On-line E-course: https://liveforexcellenceacademy.com/

You're Hired! Power Tactics: Job Search Strategies That Work

(This is an e-box set containing the complete content of Resume Tactics, Job Interview Preparation & Leveraging Your Network)

E-book: https://powertactics.online/

Power Networking for Shy People: How to Network Like a Pro

E-book & Paperback: https://powernetworkingforshypeople.ca

The Savvy Emcee: How to be a Dynamic Master of Ceremonies

E-book: https://thesavvyemcee.com

Working With Words: How to Add Life to Your Oral Presentations

E-book & Paperback: https://workingwithwordsbook.com/

Blow Your Own Horn! Personal Branding for Business Professionals

E-book & Paperback: https://blowyourownhorn.online/

If you have found this book and program to be helpful, please leave us a warm review wherever you purchased your book.

CONNECT WITH US

Visit us on the web at https://elderathome.ca

Follow us on Facebook https://www.facebook.com/agingwithhelp for a source of informational, thought-provoking articles to help you in your role as a family caregiver.

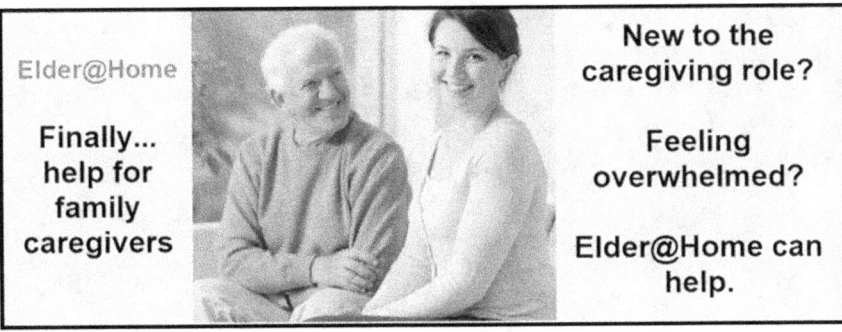

www.ingramcontent.com/pod-product-compliance
Lightning Source LLC
Chambersburg PA
CBHW070043120526
44589CB00035B/2276